THE 90-SECOND FITNESS SOLUTION

THE
90-SECOND
FITNESS SOLUTION

The Most Time-Efficient Workout Ever
for a Healthier, Stronger, Younger You

PETE CERQUA

with

ALISA BOWMAN

ATRIA BOOKS

New York   London   Toronto   Sydney

ATRIA BOOKS
A Division of Simon & Schuster, Inc.
1230 Avenue of the Americas
New York, NY 10020

Copyright © 2008 by Peter Cerqua

All rights reserved, including the right to reproduce this book or portions thereof in any form whatsoever. For information address Atria Books Subsidiary Rights Department, 1230 Avenue of the Americas, New York, NY 10020.

First Atria Books hardcover edition January 2009

ATRIA BOOKS and colophon are trademarks of Simon & Schuster, Inc.

For information about special discounts for bulk purchases, please contact Simon & Schuster Special Sales at 1-800-456-6798 or business@simonandschuster.com.

Manufactured in the United States of America

10 9 8 7 6 5 4 3 2 1

Library of Congress Cataloging-in-Publication Data
Cerqua, Pete.
   The 90-second fitness solution: the most time-efficient workout ever for a healthier, stronger, younger you / Pete Cerqua with Alisa Bowman.   —1st ed.
       p.   cm.
   Includes bibliographical references.
   1. Physcial fitness. 2. Reducing exercises. 3. Weight loss. I. Bowman, Alisa. II. Title. III. Title: The ninety-second fitness solution.
   RA781.C35   2008
   613.7—dc22   2008033893

ISBN-13: 978-1-4165-6648-9
ISBN-10:   1-4165-6648-1

For my sons, Nicholas and Jack.
You're my proudest achievements.

CONTENTS

AUTHOR'S NOTE

Why this book? I'll tell you why. Your life is already too complicated. On top of shuttling your kids to soccer, working ten-plus hours a day, caring for aging parents, and everything else, you don't need a complicated and time-consuming fitness and nutrition plan. On this plan, you eliminate complication. You save time. You get results by doing less rather than more. By doing my unique 90-second sets, you'll be able to shrink your workout from the usual forty to sixty minutes to just three. That's right. That's not a typo. My shortest workout lasts just three minutes. Do it five times a week—for a total of fifteen weekly minutes of exercise—and you'll drop a dress size in eight weeks! Interested? I thought so.

Most diet and exercise programs do the opposite. You start something and get no results, so a trainer tells you to add more. That doesn't work, so a popular diet tells you to cut out a food group. The next thing you know, a third of your week is devoted to starving and sweating. Who has time for that?

I'd like you to spend a third of your week getting and having a life. I don't want you to spend it in the gym, and I don't want you to spend it dreaming about the foods you can't eat. That's why you're going to buy this book. You will because you want that third of your week back too.

You'll get it back by eliminating everything you don't need. In its place, you'll add an efficient program that makes sense, one that will simplify not only your diet and exercise program but also your life. This program answers the questions, "How much can I get away with?" and "How little do I have to do?" I'm going to give you advice like:

This is all you need.

Don't do more than you have to.

If you can do the job in one rep, then why do two?

If you don't want to sweat or change your clothes, then don't do either.

My program is backed by second, third, and fourth concurring opinions. I have hundreds of reputable studies to support my recommendations. The proof, however, isn't in my background as a trainer and it's not really in the studies. It's in the program. You can prove to yourself right now in the bookstore that this program works. Look for the home workout on page 38 and check out the Wall Sit. Do it right here in the store. Pretty challenging, right? How much time did it just take you to fry your legs? Ninety seconds. Now buy the book, go home, and do the other *half* of the workout (the other 90 seconds) and you're done! Really. I'm not joking. In three minutes, you'll make over your workout, your body, and your life.

I want to hear from you about your success with this program. E-mail me at info@90secondfitnesssolution.com and tell me your story. I'd love to include your story of success on my Web site.

Yours in strength and health,

INTRODUCTION

Create the 90-Second Body

I'm going to take a wild guess about the nature of your life. If you are like the thousands of women I've trained during the past twenty-three years, then you probably sleep five to six hours at night, waking early to commute thirty or more minutes to a job where you spend eight or more hours before commuting back home again. If you have a spouse and kids, you do 70 percent of the parenting and housework. Make that 80 percent. If you're single, you're out every night—socializing, volunteering, taking night classes, you name it. No matter your age, marital status, or career, you don't know the concept of spare time. Sleep? Cutting back on it is how you find time to write thank-you notes and balance your checkbook, not to mention make yourself that hot breakfast that everyone tells you is so good for you.

Exercise? You'd love to, right after you catch up on your sleep and figure out how to find an extra forty-five minutes every day. Supplements? You've been meaning to buy about thirty or so different brands that you've heard might give you more energy, but you haven't had time to get to the health food store. Stress relief? You'd love some, but the idea of finding twenty spare minutes to practice meditation, deep breathing,

You bought this book because you have no time to spare. I get that. Because I'm assuming you are too hurried to read this book word for word, I've provided you with speed-reading notes in each chapter. If you don't have time to read the entire introduction, this is what you need to know:

› You can drop a dress size, lose ten pounds, cinch your belt a notch tighter, and dramatically improve your health in *just eight weeks.*

› You'll do it by spending less time exercising, less time preparing food, and less time trying to balance it all. In fact, you can do it with just fifteen minutes of weekly exercise.

› You'll accomplish more—stronger bones, more energy, a better mood, a firmer body, greater peace of mind—with less time, less money, and less overall complication. That's what the 90-Second Fitness Solution is all about.

or progressive muscle relaxation stresses you out. Healthful eating? If only someone would invent a healthful frozen dinner and convenience food diet. (Well, someone has, and it's me!)

What if I told you that you don't have to trade off your personal sanity to create a healthier, stronger, sexier, younger you? What if I told you that you could firm up, lose weight, strengthen your bones, reduce joint stiffness, boost your mood and energy levels, improve your memory, and create glowing skin in less time than it takes you to pack your kid's school lunch box? Would you sign up? I bet you would, and it's true. With the 90-Second Fitness Solution you will:

› Drop a dress size and tighten your belt one notch in eight weeks. If you currently suffer from joint pain or back pain, you can expect your pain to resolve within this period of time.

> Firm your body and burn fat with as few as fifteen *weekly* minutes of exercise. That's right. That's weekly exercise, not daily exercise.

> Eat all of the world's healthiest foods without counting a single calorie or carb, reading labels, or cooking complicated recipes. My plan is so easy and so simple that you'll never need to grocery-shop with a list again.

> Bolster your health with just three supplements—widely available online, at your local convenience store, and even at Wal-Mart—for a cost of just $10 a month.

> Ease your mind with simple space-saving tactics, such as spending five minutes a few times a week to declutter your home or office.

Call it a gimmick if you'd like, but don't tell me it doesn't work until you try it. I'm confident that you'll be amazed by your results. Most of my clients were like you. They were leery when I told them about my plan. They didn't believe so little exercise could do *anything*. They didn't believe that they could stop counting calories and carbs. They accused me of blasphemy when I encouraged them to eat an avocado or two for lunch or dinner rather than make a gourmet meal with numerous side dishes.

Then they tried it. Their bodies got tighter and smaller. Their bones got stronger. They slept more deeply, handled stress better, and felt the best they had in years. Then they told fifty friends, who came to me feeling just as leery. I eventually made believers out of them, and I'll make one out of you too.

I only ask for you to have an open mind and to *try it*. Go ahead and grumble as much as you want about how you think a program this short and this easy could never actually work. Go ahead and tell yourself that you're only going to try it for two weeks. Moan and groan behind my back as much as you want, but *do* try it.

Once you try it, you'll see. You won't stop. The initial two weeks will turn into four and then into eight and eventually into a year and then the rest of your life.

PETE'S SOLUTION FOR A HURRIED LIFE

I designed the 90-Second Fitness Solution primarily for my female clients, the ones who desperately needed and wanted all of the benefits of a fit and healthy lifestyle but who did not have the time, inclination, or lifestyle to fit in everything that the so-called experts recommended. It seemed every week a busy woman would call and tell me that she wanted to boost her metabolism, firm muscle, lift her mood, sleep more deeply, strengthen her bones, improve her health, boost her energy, and burn off that apple pie she'd eaten the night before. She'd tell me that she'd already gone to gyms and worked out nearly every day with personal trainers. She'd purchased any number of contraptions advertised on television. She'd tried most of the available exercise videos and DVDs, and she'd hated every minute of it.

She'd tell me:

1. "I don't want to sweat."
2. "I don't want to wear a leotard or expensive exercise clothes."
3. "I don't want to spend an hour every day working out."

She wanted a sensible plan she could stick with, one she would not abandon by January 15. (Most of my new clients come to me on January 2.)

It got me thinking. Just how much exercise do people really need? Sure, the government and the so-called experts recommend ninety daily minutes, but do people *really* need that much? Is there a way to make one exercise session so intense and so effective that someone could get the benefits of ninety minutes of exercise in just a few minutes?

I decided to find out.

I knew strength training—and not cardio—was the most efficient way to lose weight and get healthy. (If you're not convinced, wait until chapter 1. After reading it,

VERONICA WEISMANN

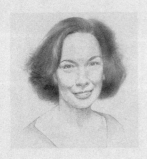

When I started training with Pete, I weighed 247 pounds. My blood pressure was 145 over 120 and my blood sugar was high enough to earn me a prediabetes diagnosis. The excess weight put pressure on my joints, creating so much back pain that I could barely move.

My husband accompanied me to my first appointment with Pete. I was frightened. I figured that I was going to be the fattest and the oldest person (at the time I was in my late forties) in the gym. I also wasn't completely convinced that Pete's workout was going to work. In fact, I thought it was impossible that one short, weekly workout was going to help me lose nearly a hundred pounds. He has since made me a believer. As I tell all of my friends, one workout with Pete is equal to six workouts somewhere else.

At first I went just once a month. I was worried that doing anything more would hurt my back. Somehow I managed to lose ten pounds. Six months later, after I was convinced that my back pain had resolved, I began training once a week, and I also began taking Pete's eating suggestions seriously.

Instead of skipping meals (my usual weight-loss tactic up to that point), I began eating regular meals, especially breakfast. I reorganized my kitchen, stocking my shelves with high-fiber, whole foods and getting rid of tempting foods that I didn't want to eat. I stopped getting my coffee at a café to avoid the temptation of eating one of those huge, six-hundred-calorie muffins. I began planning my meals better to avoid the temptation of coming home from work, feeling too tired to cook, and consequently ordering a pizza. Finally, I stopped celebrating with food. Instead of going out to eat to celebrate, I would go for a walk or go shopping.

It took me a year and a half, but I did it. I got down to my goal of 150. As the weight dropped, my health improved. My blood pressure, cholesterol, and blood sugar are now all normal. As I lost weight and got stronger, I transformed. The more I strengthened my body with Pete, the more I wanted to move and exercise. I now love to work out. I can't stand it if I can't get to the gym to move my body.

It's now been ten years since I lost the weight. Last year I tried the indoor climbing wall at a resort and was able to go higher than two people who were in their twenties! The last time I had my bone density checked, my doctor told me I had the bones of an eighteen-year-old. Pete's program absolutely, positively works. I'm living proof.

JOLYNN BACA

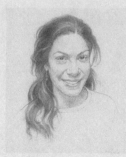

I started training with Pete in September 2006 to learn his method and eventually work for him as a fitness trainer. I'd already been teaching aerobics for five years, and I thought I was in pretty good shape. I was amazed that in just fifteen minutes Pete had me shaking, breathless, and exhausted, and all from moving at a really slow pace, or, in some cases, not moving at all. I'm five feet, a hundred pounds, and Pete had me leg pressing four hundred pounds! That's something I never thought I'd be able to do.

I noticed changes in my body right away. When I switched from my summer wardrobe to my winter wardrobe, I noticed that my winter clothes fit me dramatically differently. I was more sculpted in certain places. I started running this year, and thanks to Pete's program, I've been able to do it pain free, despite an old knee injury from my tap-dancing days.

Now I'm training clients with Pete's 90-Second Sets. Many people, at first, can't believe how much we charge for such a short session. I always tell them that this is about quality and not quantity. It really does work, and being able to get it in within such a short period of time is ideal, especially for women who are usually so overextended. Many of the women I train are amazed when I tell them that I practice what I preach. They always assume that lifting heavy weights will make them bulky. I ask, "Do you think I look bulky?" They never do.

you'll donate that old treadmill to charity.) I decided to create the most efficient strength training workout ever. I first recommended my female clients do the same weight lifting workouts men had been doing for years to build muscle and shrink fat, but when women did these eight-to-twelve-repetition, multiset weight-room workouts, they not only complained about the full hour they spent in the gym, but they also built more muscle than they wanted. They got big and bulky and, as a result, stopped exercising.

I next tried the popular approach of using a high number of repetitions with light resistance. That didn't work either. These workouts lasted thirty to forty-five minutes, and they were a complete waste of time. After spending hours working out, the women I trained lost no weight or inches. Some even gained weight. I then tried everything from one set per exercise to ten sets per exercise, ten-minute workouts to two-hour workouts, six days per week to just one day per week. I had heard about a new workout for body-builders that involved lifting very heavy weights very slowly. The problem was that it made bodybuilders smaller rather than bigger. It got me thinking.

I began experimenting with slow-speed lifting. I asked women to do ten-second rep-etitions (taking ten seconds to lift the weight, ten seconds to lower). Not only was this unproductive but it was also too boring! I asked them to do longer sets, as long as five minutes. I tried all kinds of combinations. After much trial and error, I discovered the perfect amount of time for a set was ninety seconds. I also arrived at another discovery: the speed of the movement didn't matter. What really shaped up people in record time was not slow lifting but completely *stopping* and holding the weight in key positions.

I went on to experiment with healthy eating. I'd read the research. I knew what foods were healthy and which ones were not. I knew, for instance, that trans fats, cer-tain additives, too much salt, environmental contaminants, too much sugar, and too much starch shortened a person's life span, muddled thinking, caused depression, raised risk for disease, and, yes, even encouraged weight gain. I also knew that antioxidants, fiber, omega-3 fatty acids, and lean protein promoted optimal health, energy, mood, and body weight. The question was this: How does a woman with an insane life find a way to consume all of the good foods and few of the bad ones without adding a layer of complication and stress to her life? I found my answer in my Real Food Diet. As you will soon learn, if you stick with real foods 95 percent of the time, you'll automatically consume the right balance of antioxidants, healthful fats, and other health-promoting nutrients.

I also uncovered many other nutritional surprises that many of my female clients found quite liberating. Do you feel guilty about your nightly glass of wine because you've heard it packs on the abdominal fat? Rest easy. When I studied the research, I discovered that moderate drinking not only promoted good health, but it also led to a slimmer waistline. The same was true for many fatty foods such as whole eggs, avocados, nuts, and peanut butter. These delicious foods could all be a part of both a healthy diet and a weight-loss diet. Most important, these delicious foods are among the most convenient foods to prepare. Talk about removing complication and stress!

I also experimented with supplements, wondering: *Do people really need to take thirty expensive pills a day?* I found my answer in the research. You only need three to five supplements. That's it. Case closed. See chapter 4 for the proof.

Finally, I took a look at lifestyle factors. I wanted to find ways to boost mood, reduce stress, and improve sleep quality, again, without adding a stressful layer of complication. I did that too.

Shorten your workout
Simplify your eating
Save money on supplements
Stress-proof your life

What else could you ask for in a fitness plan? I've now trained thousands of clients with the 90-Second Fitness Solution. They range from teenagers to retirees in their eighties. They include superbly gifted athletes and people with special problems such as heart disease, Parkinson's, scoliosis, and osteoporosis. They are women like Veronica, age sixty. She came to me with back problems so bad, her husband, Ron, had to walk her into the gym and help me get her through her session. She lost a hundred pounds by exercising just fifteen minutes a week with me. Read her story on page xv.

How about Staci? This thirtysomething client was a very active young lady and a personal trainer on top of that, but she would occasionally get sidelined with crippling back spasms and could never get the tight body she always wanted. She thought I was crazy after I told her that she needed to lift heavy weights to fix her back and tighten her body. Staci added fifteen minutes a week with me and then came to work for me, she liked it so much. After working for me for three years, she moved to Virginia, and Jolynn took her place. Read Jolynn's story on page xvi.

Throughout the pages of *The 90-Second Fitness Solution*, you'll read about Jolynn, Veronica, and many other women like them. Read their stories. Peruse the research. I've provided it all for you in the following pages and in an extensive bibliography at the end of the book. Most important, try the program. What do you have to lose? Body fat, bad health, stiff joints, and fatigue, that's what. You already bought the book. Get your money's worth. Try it. You won't be disappointed.

PART I
THE SCIENCE

CHAPTER 1

The Four Secrets
of Success

Did everything I say in the introduction go against everything you've learned or read about fitness and wellness? Please read on. I promise I will explain it all. Throughout the pages of this book—and particularly in this chapter—I hope to prove to you that this program works. I'm going to prove it to you with science, with studies, with testimonials, and with results. You'll even experience some of those results by the end of this chapter. Really, I'm not kidding. By the end of the chapter—after you've discovered the four components of the 90-Second Fitness Solution—it's my hope that I will have provided you with enough facts, figures, and research to convince you that my program isn't just short and simple. It's wickedly effective too.

THE FIRST SECRET OF SUCCESS:
SHORTEN YOUR WORKOUT

My 90-Second Sets compress an hour or more of exercise into as few as three minutes, and they do this with strength training. Three minutes of cardio isn't going to get you

The 90-Second Fitness Solution includes four components:

> **THE SHORTEST-EVER WORKOUT:** You'll use my 90-Second Sets to firm up, boost your metabolism, and build strength with as few as fifteen weekly minutes of exercise.

> **THE SIMPLEST-EVER EATING PLAN:** You'll live longer, live better, and lose weight without measuring foods, counting calories, or doing math of any kind. You can even do it while eating the same basic repertoire of foods day after day after day.

> **THE LEAST EXPENSIVE–EVER SUPPLEMENT PLAN:** You can ensure good health with as few as three supplements, at a cost of less than $10 a month.

> **THE LOWEST-STRESS LIFESTYLE PLAN:** You can reduce stress, sleep better, and feel happier in fewer than five minutes a day.

results. Three minutes of yoga or Pilates won't cut it. Three minutes of stretching—nothing.

Three minutes of strength training gets you a lot. You might not rank "strength" high on your list of things you need right now, but I can guarantee you that a stronger body will change your life in more ways that you can ever imagine. Before starting my program, for instance, one of my clients needed her doorman to help her lug her son's hockey bag from her apartment to the car. After fewer than three months, this 105-pound woman no longer needed her doorman's help. She just tossed the bag over her shoulder and carried it herself.

Imagine what your life would be like if you did not need help to install an air conditioner in a window, place a five-gallon water jug on your water cooler, or carry boxes full of charity donations to the car.

If you play sports, my 90-Second Sets will improve your game. You'll hit longer drives on the golf course and harder serves on the tennis court. You'll have more strength and stamina for yoga and Pilates. Most important, you'll be able to do any of these recreational activities without getting injured.

You'll live longer and healthier too. Strength training has been shown to reduce cholesterol and blood pressure and to normalize blood glucose. It boosts mood and energy and it strengthens your bones. Studies now show that strength training beats cardio for reducing the risk of heart disease and diabetes, lowering blood pressure, normalizing blood sugar, and reducing cholesterol.

Most important, you'll burn fat and lose weight. The lean muscle tissue that you build through strength training will boost your metabolism. Each pound of muscle burns thirty-five to fifty daily calories just to maintain itself. Most adults lose between five to seven pounds of muscle each decade, which slows metabolic rate by up to 5 percent and results in a gain of fifteen pounds of fat during the same decade. Strength training reverses this muscle wasting. Most women can add back three pounds of their lost muscle within eight weeks of starting a strength training program. Just three more pounds of muscle is enough to speed the metabolism by 7 percent, increasing the number of calories burned by 15 percent. That will reduce your body by a half a dress size to a dress size *even if you do nothing to change your eating habits.* Really, I'm not making this up. In one study completed at Tufts University, adults who strength-trained shrank four pounds of fat within three months, even if they consumed 15 percent more calories!

So now you know why strength training—and not cardio or stretching—is the most effective and efficient way to get fit and healthy. Now, let's talk about the unique specifics of the 90-Second Fitness Solution by dispelling a number of strength training myths.

SARA WILFORD

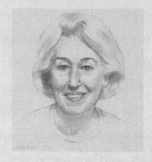

I'm seventy-five and I have severe osteoarthritis. I was trying to do everything I could to slow the progression. My doctor told me that strength training might help, and a friend suggested Pete. Time is a huge factor for me, but she told me that I could do his workout in just fifteen minutes a week. I just couldn't believe it. I'd never heard of anything that could make a difference in that amount of time, but I decided to make an appointment.

Pete started me very slowly on a series of machines. To my amazement, I began to build upper-body strength. Recently I went to the internist for some blood work, and the nurse looked at me and said, "Sara, you've got muscles." I said, "I do?" They aren't huge but they are firm and they are strong. The strength is important to me because of my knee. I can now use my arms to pull myself up a flight of steps. It gives me a sense of power and it's kept me mobile.

I was so impressed with Pete that I started taking my husband, age eighty, with me to my sessions. My husband has always been fit, but after I had been training with Pete for a while, I could tell that my husband was not lifting weights correctly. Now we train with Pete together. Going to Pete gave him more power in his upper body too. He looks terrific.

MYTH 1:
YOU NEED CARDIO TO LOSE WEIGHT

I'd like to tackle this myth by telling you a story. I met a woman at a party one of my clients was hosting. I walked up while she was complaining about her weight. My client introduced me to her, saying, "This is my personal trainer, the guy I was telling you about."

Without much prodding, she began to tell me her tale of woe. As a relatively new lawyer, her responsibilities had risen dramatically. She averaged sixty weekly hours at the office. On top of that she was engaged to be married and was planning a wedding. At five-foot two and 120 pounds, she didn't need to lose weight, but she worried that the stress of her job coupled with her other responsibilities would soon catch up with her. Her solution was to train to run the New York City marathon. Her routine was to run three to five times per week and hit the weights twice per week. The weight work consisted of light weights and high reps "to burn more calories." (Sound familiar? You may have tried something like this yourself.)

She followed this plan religiously. Six months later she found herself at a "buff" and built 140 pounds. She laughed as she told me that her fiancé was just as repulsed by her new physique as she was. I suggested she do one strength workout with me per week, one high-intensity cardio workout, and one thirty-minute walk while listening to relaxing music. If she felt as if she hadn't done enough, she could add a yoga or Pilates class to her schedule. She also took the supplements I recommended and followed my Real Food Diet. It worked. She got back down to 120 pounds and was smaller, tighter, stronger, and healthier.

So you see, as much as you've heard that you need to "burn off those calories" and "melt off that fat," cardio just doesn't cut it when it comes to slimming down. Strength training is the most effective way to lose weight. Cardio doesn't even run a close second. Strength training works because you get a triple calorie-burning benefit for every workout. You burn calories during your workout as you lift and lower the weight. If you've tried my workouts by now, then you know that they get your heart rate up. That means your metabolic rate is up too.

Now, taken head to head, cardio probably burns more calories during a workout than even the most intense strength training, but the real benefit of strength training happens after the workout. For about forty-eight hours after each session, your metabolic rate remains elevated as your body builds and replaces lean muscle tissue. Now for the triple burn that no amount of cardio can provide: for every pound of lean muscle tissue you build through strength training, you speed up your metabolism by thirty-five to fifty calories a day.

MYTH 2:
YOU NEED CARDIO TO STAY HEALTHY

Strength training provides a much bigger health gain for your exercise buck. For example, you've probably heard that exercise helps prevent diabetes, right? Well, which type of exercise do you think helps more, cardio or strength training? Most people think cardio, because they've been told for years that this is the type of exercise that improves health. Strength training gets you strong, they think, and cardio gets you healthy. It's just not true, and I have research to prove it. A team of researchers at the Department of Diabetes and Rheumatology at Wilhelminenspital in Vienna, Austria, asked eleven men and eleven women with type 2 diabetes (the type that used to be called "adult onset" because it didn't usually develop until adulthood) to take part in either a four-month strength training program or a four-month cardiovascular exercise program. The strength training group exercised two to three times a week. The cardio group started with fifteen daily minutes of exercise and worked up to thirty daily minutes.

Four months later, who was healthier? The strength trainers. They hadn't walked a single step (with the exception of to and from their cars and mailboxes and to and from the gym), yet they experienced a significant drop in hemoglobin A1c (a measure of average blood glucose over three months and the most important indicator of metabolic health). The cardio group? They saw no improvement in A1c. That's right. Nada.

Here's why. Stronger muscles take up and burn blood sugar more readily, reducing your risk of diabetes and stabilizing blood sugar levels 24/7. Cardio? It helps too, but only in the twenty-four hours after a session. One strength training session per week improves blood sugar control around the clock. Three weekly cardio sessions improve it only three days out of the week.

What about other metabolic factors? Oh, yes, the researchers measured those too.

GOT STRENGTH?

Check out the three illustrations depicting Sally's aging body. Which Sally do you want to resemble? I'm guessing it's Sally #1. She's 25 years old. At 5'2", 120 pounds, her body composition is 18% body fat. This means that she has only 21.6 pounds of fat. No wonder she looks so good.

What happened to her? She spent her 20s and early 30s working too much, partying too much, and sitting too much. She lost 7 pounds of lean muscle mass, but she looks bigger and flabbier because she gained 22 pounds of fat.

Now, look at her at age 45. She's lost 17 pounds of muscle and gained 62 pounds of fat, even though she's eating roughly the same as she did during her 20s. That lost muscle slowed her metabolism, causing her body to stockpile the fat. Her risk of heart disease and diabetes has increased dramatically and she feels sluggish all day and doesn't sleep well at night. If she goes on a crash diet or just does aerobics, she will lose weight but a large portion of that will be muscle.

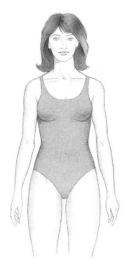 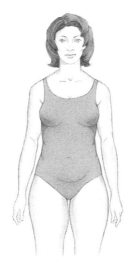 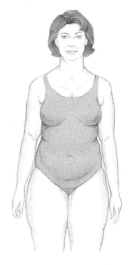

Sally #1
Age: 25
Weight: 120 pounds
Body fat: 18%

Sally #2
Age: 35
Weight: 135 pounds
Body fat: 32%

Sally #3
Age: 45
Weight: 165 pounds
Body Fat: 50%

Blood glucose levels and insulin sensitivity both improved in the strength trainers but not in the cardio exercisers. Total cholesterol dropped an average twenty-three points, the artery-clogging LDL type dropped fourteen points, and triglycerides (a type of blood fat that raises risk for heart disease, especially in women) dropped an average seventy-nine points in the strength training group. The cardio group? Again, they got nothing. The strength trainers also improved their good HDL cholesterol by five points, and, you guessed it, the cardio group saw no change.

That thirty minutes of daily cardio sure is sounding more and more like a waste of good time to me.

Now you know what two to three weekly sessions of strength training can do in people with diabetes. What if you're healthy and just don't want to get sick? Can a few weekly strength training sessions keep you healthy, even if you do no or very little cardio? By now, you should already know what I'm going to say, but I'll indulge your curiosity. Yes, they can. In a study of fifty-four healthy women between the ages of thirty-five and fifty, women who strength-trained just twice a week without doing *any* cardio got even healthier in just fifteen weeks. Their insulin, glucose, and IGF-1 (also known as insulin-like growth factor, which raises risk for cancer) all dropped.

Okay, now if you've been following the research and are up on your health reading, then you probably think you can still stump me. You might be thinking: *But Pete, what about mood?* Cardio is a great mood booster. Yep, you're right, it is. Cardio boosts levels of neuropeptides in the brain that boost mood and reduce stress. Know what? So does strength training. A ten-week study by Harvard researchers of thirty-two depressed seniors determined that three weekly strength training sessions significantly reduced depression, improved quality of life and social function, and even reduced sensations of pain.

Researchers and physicians now believe in the benefits of strength training so much that they recommend that people with congestive heart failure and people who are recovering from bypass surgery add strength training to their recovery programs.

I'm not trying to talk you out of cardio if you love it. If you love to run, by all means, keep running. If you love to cycle, keep cycling. I'm telling you all of this, however, so that you can feel guiltless about scrapping the cardio that you hate. You can get and stay healthy with strength training. Do cardio if you want to, not because you feel you have to.

MYTH 3:
A COMPLETE FITNESS PROGRAM INCLUDES DAILY STRETCHING

Many people believe that they absolutely need to stretch to improve sports performance, stay flexible, reduce muscle soreness, and clear the lactic acid that builds up during exercise. Let's address each of these supposed benefits one at a time.

SPORTS PERFORMANCE: Various studies have shown that *strength training* improves sports performance. For example, in a Greek study of eighteen soccer players, twice-weekly strength training improved soccer technique, shuttle-run speed, and sprinting speed more than another group of soccer players who did not strength-train. Stretching? Results are mixed, with some showing that it may even reduce performance, particularly in runners. A United Kingdom study of thirty-four elite male distance runners, for instance, determined that the least flexible runners had the most efficient strides, meaning they used less energy as they ran compared to more flexible runners. In a Canadian review of twenty-three studies that looked into the effects of stretching on sports performance, twenty-two of the studies concluded that stretching produced no effect on muscle force or jumping height. Of four studies that looked at running speed, one found a negative effect and two found no effect.

FLEXIBILITY: Yes, daily stretching can lengthen muscles, giving you more range of motion around a joint, but so can strength training, and you need to strength-train much less often to get the same effect. In a Greek study of thirty-two seniors, strength training increased sit-and-reach flexibility (basically hamstring and back flexibility) as well as range of motion at the elbow, knee, shoulder, and hip joints. A separate Greek study of fifty-eight seniors found similar results, showing that the more intense the strength training program, the more flexible became the study's participants. That's one of the reasons I want you to lift heavy; it gets you as flexible as it gets you strong.

MUSCLE SORENESS: There are only three things that reduce muscle soreness: time, painkillers, and ice. A group of Australian researchers reviewed ten studies (all of the available studies done at that time) on the effects of stretching on muscle soreness. Whether study participants stretched before exercise or after, the activity had no effect on muscle soreness.

LACTIC ACID: Don't you need to stretch after exercise in order to work lactic acid out of your muscles? I'll address this one by quoting Australian researchers who published a review about exercise recovery in the medical journal *Sports Medicine*: "After high intensity exercise, rest alone will return blood lactate to baseline levels well within the normal time period between training sessions."

INJURY PREVENTION: Strength training has been shown to reduce falls in the elderly, prevent broken bones induced by osteoporosis (the bone-thinning disease), and reduce the progression of and pain from osteoarthritis. It also reduces sports-induced injuries. Core strength—in the abdomen and back—has even been shown to reduce injuries in firefighters by 62 percent. Stretching? It *might* help, especially if one leg is tighter than the other or if muscle tightness in one area of your body is throwing off your posture.

So you see, it's not that stretching provides no benefits but that strength training provides *all of the same* benefits in much less time. As with cardio, I'm not telling you to forgo stretching if you love it. Many of my clients love their weekly yoga classes because of how this form of exercise makes them feel. If you love it, do it. If you hate it, don't.

MYTH 4:
WOMEN NEED LIGHT RESISTANCE AND LOTS OF REPS

Let me tackle this myth by telling you a story. In the book *One More Rep* by John Little and Robert Wolff, the authors describe one of the workout routines used by a champion bodybuilder, Flex Wheeler. For his shoulders, Flex did four sets of fifteen reps of side laterals using only twenty-five-pound dumbbells (which is very light for him). For added size to his shoulders, he added reps and took those twenty-five-pound dumbbells up to sixty reps per set! This is typical of what many top bodybuilders would do to get that freakish "Michelin Man" look. Most women's workout routines resemble a version of a top bodybuilder's workout. If a top bodybuilder would start doing my 90-Second Sets, he would lose his pump faster than most people lose diet willpower when they sit down to Thanksgiving dinner.

If I've learned one thing in more than twenty years of training thousands of people, it's that high-rep weight training can result in only two outcomes:

1. If the weights are too light, it does nothing at all.
2. If the weights are heavy enough to do anything, it makes you look like Flex Wheeler.

But, you're thinking, women can't add bulk. At least, that's what all the experts keep saying. Well, that's a bunch of hogwash. Yes, women don't have the testosterone levels to add as much muscle as *male* bodybuilders do. (Okay, so I was exaggerating just a little when I said you'd end up looking like Flex Wheeler.) Women *can* add bulk, though. A woman with a ten-inch-circumference bicep is not going to be able to double the size of her bicep (at least not without some pharmaceutical help), but she can certainly add an inch of size. I don't know too many women who want to grow

WENDY COHEN

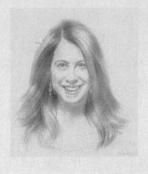

To get in shape and to look good, I started lifting weights almost twenty years ago, when I was twenty-four. As I got older, however, the strength training took on a new meaning. I didn't want to get old. I wanted to stay strong and healthy, and I knew weight training was the only way to get those results.

I haven't always had the best results with strength training, though. Certain approaches bulked me up, making me look awful. Other programs didn't bulk me up, but they required I spend an hour at the gym twice a week. I just don't have that kind of time.

Then I heard about Pete. I started his program, and now I have extra time each week to take a yoga class. The yoga is a gift. Now I feel fit and healthy, and exercise hasn't taken over my life to get me that way.

Of course, I want to look good, but I mostly go because I want to be healthy and strong and I don't want to make getting healthy and strong a daily, time-consuming project. Pete's program gives me the same results I got in other strength training programs, but in much less time. When I go to Pete, I know I'm getting the job done. It's such a great feeling to leave his place and know that I'm done for the week. It's a fabulous feeling.

their biceps by an inch. That's not sexy in a spaghetti strap, but that's what happens when you go low weight, high rep. To lose inches, you need to lift heavy. With my approach, you'll gain strength without adding bulk. You'll get *stronger* as your body grows *smaller.*

Take Wendy. Wendy was in her midforties when she came to me. Wendy knew she needed to exercise to age gracefully. She knew that strength training was the way to go. With a hectic schedule and limited information, she'd hired a personal trainer. Her trainer put her through the standard three sets of twelve reps on about a dozen exercises. Even though Wendy was getting stronger and healthier from her workouts, her arms were getting bigger than her husband's.

A friend of Wendy's was already getting great results with me. Wendy liked how her friend looked, so she decided to give my method a try. She was skeptical, of course. "I bulk up too easily," she said. I said, "No problem. I'll make you twice as strong and get rid of that pumped look you're carrying around."

In eight weeks, Wendy got rid of the bulk! Now twice as strong, she can wear spaghetti straps without feeling self-conscious about her arms. Read her complete story on page 14.

MYTH 5:
YOU MUST WORK OUT FOR FORTY-FIVE MINUTES OR LONGER TO GET RESULTS

As I was developing this program, I watched people work out. I timed their sets and their rest periods and I asked them about their results. I watched as people worked out for as long as ninety minutes. Despite the amount of time they were in the gym, they actually spent most of the time talking, looking in the mirror, drinking water, resting between sets, and setting up their equipment. In terms of actual exercise, most only lifted for a total of nine minutes. That's ridiculous, I thought. It didn't seem like an efficient way to get into shape.

My workouts do the opposite. They include between two and seven exercises, all of which take 90 seconds to complete. You do only one set of each exercise, and then you're done. It's incredibly efficient. My shortest workout takes just three minutes to complete but it gets you just as strong as that ninety-minute workout.

What? You don't believe me? Most people don't.

I'd like to prove it to you the same way I prove to it people I meet at parties.

Partygoers get very upset when I tell them that one rep is better than twelve, and that one set is better than three. I prove my point by asking, "Who can do the most push-ups?" A man will usually step forward and claim that he can do twenty-five or more. I ask him, "What do you think is more challenging, twenty-five push-ups or one push-up?" It's a trick question, but it always generates the same response. He says twenty-five. So I follow up with, "If you can do twenty-five push-ups, then you can do just one, right?" He puffs out his chest and says that one rep is cake. He looks at me as if I'm an idiot.

Then I say, "Let's see if you can do one rep Pete's way." I coach him through the lowering phase of the push-up, making him stop and hold each inch down for ten seconds. When he gets to the bottom, I tell him to start pushing back up, holding each inch. Most guys can't, and the ones who can are bright red in the cheeks and breathing heavily. Either way, I usually say something smart-assed like, "If you can do twenty-five reps, why couldn't you do just one of mine?"

Now, I want to do the same with you. I'd like you to get on the floor and do the "Prove it to Yourself" exercise described on page 17.

How do you feel? It was pretty challenging, wasn't it? I bet it was! Are you starting to understand how this works? It works because you are making better use of your time. Can you see how this shortens your workout? If you do a traditional weight lifting workout, you'll do about ten reps per exercise, spending about fifteen seconds per set. You'll do twelve different exercises, three sets of ten reps each. That adds up to thirty-six sets. Between each set, you must rest and recover, usually for about two minutes. Do the math and you will find, as I have, that thirty-six sets will take about ninety minutes, but your muscles will actually be working for only about 540 seconds, or about nine minutes. That's a lot of wasted time.

Consider the numbers on page 18. I've actually made every attempt in the following comparison to give traditional workouts their just rewards. I don't require *any* rest between sets, but I've accounted for some here, given that it takes some time to walk from one machine to another.

You're going to do a push-up Pete's way. Get on the floor in a plank position, with your arms under your chest and your legs extended.

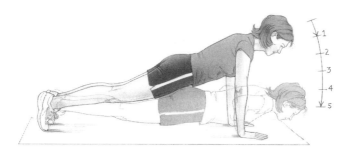

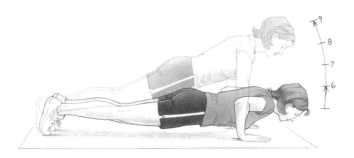

1. Lower yourself two inches and hold for ten seconds.
2. Lower yourself two more inches and hold for ten.
3. Continue lowering and holding a few inches at a time until you get to hold #5 on the accompanying illustration. Your chest should be two to four inches from the floor.
4. Then push up two inches higher and hold for ten seconds. Push up two more inches and hold for ten seconds.
5. Your arms are fully extended in the plank position. Hold for ten.

Okay, you're done. If you can get yourself off the floor, you now have Pete's permission to read on.

	PETE'S	CONVENTIONAL
Number of exercises	7	12
Number of sets	7	36
Time per set	90 sec	15 sec
Rest between sets	15 sec	2 min
Total time spent lifting weights	10½ min	9 min
Time spent in the gym	12 min	70+ min

With my approach, you are working hard every single second. My unique stopping method—what I call steps—induces a more intense muscular contraction. It gets you stronger, faster. I've seen this time and time again in training thousands of people. Studies conducted by the well-respected Wayne L. Westcott, Ph.D., fitness research director at the South Shore YMCA in Quincy, Massachusetts, have also proven this. Westcott split beginner exercisers into two groups, one lifting traditionally (spending about seven seconds per rep) and one lifting in a slower manner similar to my 90-Second Sets. The slow-moving lifters gained 50 percent more strength over ten weeks than the traditional lifters.

My 90-Second Sets are also safer because the technique minimizes momentum. You may remember from high school physics that force = mass x acceleration. If acceleration is near zero, then force is minimal even if the weight is large. Healthy mothers often hurt their backs picking up twenty-five-pound toddlers, not because the weight is too heavy, but because they try to lift the weight too abruptly. Conversely, no one ever gets injured when I ask them to go up to a wall, place their hands on it, and push as hard as they can. In fact, that's a wonderful way to build whole-body strength safely.

MYTH 6:
YOU NEED TO FAIL TO SUCCEED

Many weight loss exercise programs require you to find your edge, torturing yourself to endure as much as your body can possibly handle during each and every workout. In other words, you lift a weight over and over again until you cannot lift it a single additional time. You try to lift the final rep but can't. It's known as training to failure.

I believe in success, not failure. Not only is lifting to failure demotivating, it's unnecessary. In a study completed at the Research and Sports Medicine Center in Navarre, Spain, researchers determined that weight lifters who did not lift to failure gained just as much strength as lifters who went to failure. The ones who did not lift to failure also showed better hormonal changes after the workout, indicating that the repair and strengthening process was going more smoothly inside their bodies.

MYTH 7:
YOU NEED TO DO THE ENTIRE NAUTILUS CIRCUIT TO GET RESULTS

Most gym workouts include ten to twelve different exercises. That's why so many people at the gym carry these little pieces of paper around with them. They need to write down their workouts because they can't remember all of the exercises. Research shows that the human brain can retain only about seven pieces of information at a time. That's one reason why none of my workouts in chapter 2 contain more than seven exercises. My shortest workout includes just two.

Reason number two? Doing more than seven exercises is overkill, assuming your routine includes big exercises rather than small ones. Big exercises force your body to use many muscles at once. Small exercises zero in on just one body part—say the biceps—with a biceps curl. Most of my 90-Seconds exercises are big exercises. They require you to do special "compound" movements that stimulate more muscles throughout your body (in your abdominals, back, arms, and legs). The Plank, for example, works your arms, chest, abs, back, legs, glutes, calves, toes, hands, wrists, and neck. The Wall Sit targets your legs, butt, abdominals, and low back. These two exercises work everything from your toes to your ears.

To get an idea of the difference between big and small exercises, I'd like you to get back on the floor. Yes, that's right. Right now. Do the "Prove It to Yourself" exercise on page 21 and then come back to the book. Did you see the difference? The big exercise did more than the small exercise in the same amount of time.

I'm not saying that small exercises are worthless. I even include a few of them in my routines, especially for the body areas like the abs, which so many women want to sculpt. I don't include many, though, because I don't believe any woman should do more than she needs to, to look and feel great.

MYTH 8:
YOU NEED TO TRAIN A LOT TO STAY HEALTHY

This concept of move, move, and move some more stems from research done in the 1980s. A Harvard study published in the *New England Journal of Medicine* in 1986 analyzed the exercise habits and health outcomes of 17,000 Harvard alumni, showing that the men who were healthiest and lived the longest were exercising off about 2,000 calories a week by walking, gardening, and competing in sports. The researchers concluded that 2,000 calories per week of exercise was enough to add two years to your life.

Sounds like an open-and-shut case, doesn't it? Harvard's right. Pete's wrong. Skip

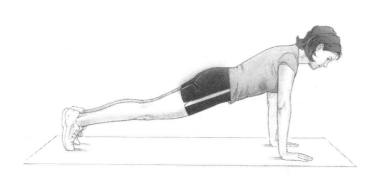

I'm sorry, but it has to be done. I need you back on the floor in a plank position. I know your arms are still shaking from the push-up, but I promise to get you in and out of the plank quickly. Place your palms on the floor under your chest with your arms extended, as shown, and extend your legs. Keep your hips up; don't allow them to sink down. Don't move. At first, you'll feel this in your arms and probably in your chest. The longer you hold, however, you'll see that you're also feeling it in your abs, back, legs, and butt. In just one exercise you're getting a total body workout, and you didn't even move a muscle!

Now let's do the opposite. Flip over, lie on your back with your knees bent. Place your hands behind your head and elbows out to the sides. Crunch up and hold. Where do you feel it? Your abs, right? Do you feel anything happening in your legs, arms, back, or chest? I didn't think so. This is an example of an isolation exercise. It zeros in on and works just one area of the body. Okay, you're done. Go ahead and crawl back to your couch and resume reading where you left off.

your short strength training session and get on the treadmill and walk or run twenty miles a week to burn off that 2,000 calories. (Ouch! It hurts me just thinking about it.)

Not so fast. You know what's wrong with this research? First, the 1980s was the

Ask Pete

Q Can I lose weight faster by eating less and then start exercising once I reach my goal weight?

A You already know where that will lead you. You'll eventually hit a plateau. You'll get hungry, suffer intense cravings, and eventually return to your old ways. The weight comes back with interest. Numerous studies show that 90 percent of dieters who do not exercise typically regain everything they lose within several months after they stop dieting. When you lose weight by dieting alone, about one-quarter of the weight you lose comes from muscle protein and not from your fat tissue. This slows your metabolism, increasing the likelihood that you'll regain the weight. The National Weight Control Registry—the largest study of individuals who have successfully lost a lot of weight and kept it off—has determined that regular exercise is the *only* solution for lasting weight loss.

height of the low-fat craze. People were consuming as much as 80 or 90 percent of their calories from carbs. If you are consuming that much carbohydrate, then, yes, you need to get on the treadmill, baby, because all of that extra blood sugar needs to go somewhere. If your muscles don't burn it up for energy, then it's going to get converted to fat and come to rest inside of a fat cell. Second, this study didn't factor strength training into the equation *at all*. Strength training and its benefits were looked down upon in the 1980s. If you lifted weights, you were a bodybuilder or muscle head. In the 1980s, few women lifted weights. Both of these factors negate the Harvard study results.

Even with strength training, most people think they need to do more than they really need. Depending on which of my strength training programs you use, you will work out as often as five days a week or as infrequently as once a week. That's right. You didn't read that wrong. I said once a week.

You've probably heard that you need to strength-train three days a week. Hit the gym any less and your muscles wither away to nothing. Again, it *isn't* true.

Westcott studied three lifting strategies: three days a week, two days a week and one day a week. The participants who exercised just once a week, gained just as much strength as the ones who lifted twice a week and 82 percent as much strength as the participants who strength trained three times a week. Need more proof? Research conducted by the Research and Sports Medicine Center, Government of Navarre, Spain, has found that once-weekly strength training along with once-weekly cardio is just as effective at building strength as twice-weekly strength training along with twice-weekly cardio. You can indeed go just as far by doing half as much.

It is an iron law of training that the harder you work, the more recovery time you need. If you don't give yourself enough rest, your body does not have time to get stronger and build new muscle. Because of this law, I recommend you do my less intense home routines more often and my more intense gym routines less often.

THE SECOND SECRET OF SUCCESS:
SIMPLIFY YOUR EATING

I always interview my weight loss clients about the diets they've tried in the past. Invariably I learn that they've tried many diets and even experienced good results. The problem is that they didn't stick with them. Whenever I ask why, the answer is usually one of the following:

> I didn't have time to follow such a complicated menu plan.

> The calorie, carb, fat gram, points, etc. counting was too tedious.

> I couldn't eat my favorite foods and always felt deprived and hungry.

These problems are surmountable with the right approach to eating. Because this program dramatically boosts your metabolism with weight lifting, you won't have to drastically reduce the amount of food you put on your plate. In fact, you could probably eat between 350 and 400 *more* daily calories and maintain your weight. More important, you don't need to count anything or follow a set menu plan. You just follow my four simple rules, which include:

1. **EAT REAL FOOD.** If you focus your choices on stuff that grows in nature or eats food that grows in nature—fruit, vegetables, legumes, eggs, meat, and fish—and not on stuff that is sold in a box or bag, you will automatically consume the right number of calories and nutrients for optimal health and weight. When you eliminate many additives and preservatives common in fake foods, you bring your body back into balance, so you'll be more likely to feel full when you should feel full, preventing overeating. You'll speed up your metabolism, too, and you'll reduce cravings.

2. **EAT VEGETABLES AND LEGUMES (BEANS, PEAS, LENTILS) FIRST.** These are nature's health-promoting powerhouse foods, and they are rich in nutrients and relatively low in calories. If at every meal and snack you first turn to these foods, you'll automatically consume the right amount of fiber, vitamins, minerals, and antioxidants—without counting a single thing.

3. **DRINK REAL BEVERAGES.** For the same reasons I tell you to eat real food, I also want you to drink real beverages. You'll learn why soft drinks and many other sources of liquid calories are destroying your health and widening your waistline, and why wine, coffee, and water are all healthy and slimming options.

4. **LIMIT RED MEAT.** Yes, it's a real food, but red meat also increases inflammation and is contaminated with dioxin. Sorry, bacon lovers. I recommend it no more than once a week, *even* if you choose nitrate-free products.

That's how you'll eat for optimal health. If you want to lose weight, you'll take things a step further by periodically doing a liquid diet for a few days (to drop

CAROL STAUBI

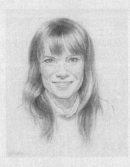

I started training with Pete because I wasn't pleased with the way I was looking. I'd tried many types of exercise plans, but nothing seemed to work over the long term. I couldn't keep it up either because of the time commitment or because it was too expensive. I work in corporate America, and I'm also in graduate school for my master's degree. I'm very busy. I needed an effective way to exercise that I could fit into my life.

I went to Pete initially for dietary advice. I told him that I am just a bad eater, that I didn't need to exercise more or differently. I met with a nutritionist on his staff who helped me find simple ways to eat more healthfully. I knew how to eat but I was just having trouble doing it. For example, I knew I needed to eat breakfast but I didn't have time to make myself a bowl of oatmeal in the morning. Instead of oatmeal, she suggested nuts and pumpkin seeds. It was great. I could just grab them on my way out the door and eat them on the go. She helped me make smarter choices at restaurants too, such as ordering the fish and chicken dishes and substituting vegetables for the starch. Once I got in the habit of simple eating, I just kept at it, coming up with my own simple strategies.

Within a couple of months, however, I realized that I couldn't change my body just by eating differently. I needed exercise too. I just wanted to get down one clothing size and I wanted to feel more confident about my problem areas. I told Pete, "If you increase my size, I am going to kill you." He just smiled and told me, "This isn't going to make you big. Trust me." I did, and he was right. I didn't get bigger. I got smaller. I've now been doing his workout for about two years. I recently visited a childhood friend in Chicago who had not seen me in years. When she saw me she said, "You're the slimmest I've ever seen you." Pete has transformed my body. Those problem areas? I no longer obsess over them. I feel better in my clothes and I feel better in my body.

pounds fast) and then eating the same repertoire of foods so that you can keep your grocery list in your head and prepare your meals by rote. You'll learn all about the whys and hows of my approach to eating in chapter 3.

THE THIRD SECRET OF SUCCESS:
SAVE MONEY ON SUPPLEMENTS

Have you been on health or diet plans that recommended hundreds of dollars in pills? It's highway robbery, in my humble opinion. Ideally, I'd recommend no supplements, but we don't live in an ideal world. Few of us eat perfectly all of the time, and modern farming practices have rendered our foods less nutritious than in the past. End result: We all need three to five pills a day. What I recommend has lots of science to back it up, and I've provided that science in chapter 4. The supplements I recommend are the same ones most physicians recommend for optimal health. They are backed by research at the Linus Pauling Institute, Harvard, and other prestigious institutions. These supplements work, and they cost you just $10 a month.

THE FOURTH SECRET OF SUCCESS:
STRESS-PROOF YOUR LIFE

So you've heard that you need to sleep eight hours at night, that you need to reduce stress, put yourself first, and take more vacations and work fewer hours. It's not bad advice, but I have a question for you. How are you doing with those goals?

I don't know many women who are sleeping more now than they did five or ten years ago. I don't know many women whose employers have doubled their vacation time or many women who take all of the vacation time that they have. That spouse and those kids are not going to disappear, and, let's face it, they won't evolve into your personal sous-chefs, massage therapists, and janitorial staff either.

It's true. Sleep *is* important. Relaxation *is* important. Happiness *is* important.

How can you have it all without doing it all too? My stress-proofing plan helps you accomplish all of these goals without stressing yourself out in the process. You can have deeper, more effective sleep without necessarily sleeping more. You can feel happier without getting a divorce or finding a spouse. You can reduce stress without adding thirty or more minutes of daily stress-reduction techniques to your already busy schedule.

You'll do it by creating more space in your life. You'll do very effective and very time-efficient tasks such as spending five minutes a few times a week reorganizing your closets, drawers, and kitchen cabinets. You'll do it by focusing on the most effective ways to calm down, boost mood, and sleep more deeply, and you'll do it by keeping track of your energetic deposits and withdrawals with Pete's Life Balance Sheet. My diet, exercise, and supplement plans will help too, as they all deepen sleep, fight fatigue, and bolster mood. You'll learn all my stress-proofing life plan in chapter 5.

WHAT ARE YOU WAITING FOR?

Whatever your goal, the 90-Second Fitness Solution will get you there.

Do you want better health? Karen Mann did. When she came to me, she was in her fifties. She had been exercising for years before she met me, and she was suffering from fibromyalgia, osteopenia, and high cholesterol. After following my instructions, she now has a lean 105-pound body and is stronger than most men. Her bones are stronger and her fibromyalgia is under control too.

Do you want a smaller body? Who doesn't? Carol Staubi was in her thirties when she came to see me. She had been doing lots of reps of light weights and she was

BULKY. When I told her that she needed to lift fewer, heavier weights more slowly, she got SMALLER and STRONGER and has stuck with me ever since. (Read Carol's story on page 25).

You can have Karen's results. You can have Carol's results. You can have *your* results. You have nothing to lose but your bad health, your flabby body, your toxic stress, and your lack of control. Get back in charge of your body, your health, your plate, and your peace of mind in the simplest way possible. Turn the page to get started.

PART II

THE
SOLUTIONS

CHAPTER 2

Shorten Your Workout

I'm guessing that I haven't made a believer out of you quite yet. I can quote you study after study, I can present you with one testimonial after another, but there's nothing like seeing and feeling the program for yourself. Let's make a deal: just try it. Give me eight weeks of your life. Give me as few as fifteen minutes a week. That's two hours of your time over eight weeks. In two hours, I am going to transform your body.

Just two hours.

What's the worst thing that could happen? You waste two hours and the about $20 you already spent on the book. If, after eight weeks, you don't like what you see, then by all means go back to the sweating, the leotards, the treadmill, and the entire hour out of your every day. Sell the book on eBay and recoup some of your investment.

What's *really* going to happen? After eight weeks, you're going to be telling your girlfriends, your spouse, and your mother about this fantastic workout that takes almost no time and delivers fantastic results. You will, because every single client I've

In this chapter, you'll find four workouts that feature my 90-Second Sets. You can do three of them at home and one at the gym:

> **HOME LEVEL 1:** Designed for beginners, I recommend you do this three-minute workout five days a week, for a total of fifteen weekly minutes.

> **HOME LEVEL 2:** Designed for people with intermediate fitness, this workout will take you roughly nine minutes. Do it up to three days a week, for a total of about twenty-seven weekly minutes.

> **HOME LEVEL 3:** Designed for fitness superstars who hate the gym, this challenging routine lasts roughly ten and a half minutes. Do it up to twice a week, for a total of about twenty-one weekly minutes.

> **GYM ROUTINE (ALL OPTIONS):** This routine takes about twelve minutes per session, depending on how quickly you move from machine to machine. Do it no more than twice a week, for a total of about twenty-four weekly minutes.

trained has done just that. I don't just train individual women. I train their entire families and social networks.

Before you dive in, I'd like you to do a little homework. I want you to make a 90-Second Scorecard. Designate a notebook, a piece of paper, or a computer file as your scorecard. Each week, write down how long you held each rep and set, along with how much weight you lifted. I've provided examples within this chapter to help you create these cards. You'll also find scorecards that you can photocopy and use starting on page 208 in chapter 7. When you see on your scorecard that you've increased your seconds or your weight, you'll build a sense of confidence and inner power that will fuel your future success. Most of the women I've trained have told me that they feel more satisfied about their workouts when this scorecard shows that they are constantly improving and getting stronger than they do seeing the pounds drop on the scale or inches shrink around their waistlines. In coming chapters, you'll learn how to use the same scorecard to keep track of your eating and lifestyle.

BUILD STRENGTH AT HOME

If you are the type of person who hates to sweat and who doesn't like to move or exert yourself, you'll fall in love with my do-it-at-home routines. These routines allow you to build strength with:

> **NO EQUIPMENT.** You'll get stronger by moving slowly or by not moving at all and by using your body weight as resistance.

> **NO EMBARRASSMENT.** If you've avoided exercise because you have thoughts like, "People will think I look ridiculous," "People will see me and wonder why such a fat person is even trying," "I already feel unattractive as it is. The last thing I need is for someone to see me in spandex," you'll love your home strength building oasis. It's as private as you want it to be.

> **NO COST.** You don't need to purchase anything to get started. You don't even need fancy clothes or sneakers.

> **NO PLANNING.** If you have a body, a wall, and a floor, you can do the routine as soon as *right now*.

> **NO FUSS.** You'll more easily make exercise a habit if you don't have to drive to and from the gym.

> **NO PAIN.** Anyone can do the home workout. I've trained women as old as eighty-five and as young as fourteen, women with knee problems, back problems, and more. It's even safe to do during pregnancy.

> › **NO SWEAT.** These routines are over before you even break a sweat. Driving to the gym, changing clothes, sweating, showering, and driving home all take a considerable amount of time. No sweat. Three minutes. Done.

FOR BEST RESULTS

You can do the home routines anywhere. As I've mentioned, all you need is a wall, a floor, and your body. You can do it barefoot or in your slippers if that suits you. My goal, however, is to make sure that you do it, you do it correctly, and you keep doing it. To that end, I recommend the following:

> › **GO GREEN.** Paint is cheap, but it can go a heck of a long way to making you happier and healthier. White walls tend to cause people to speed up their workouts, whereas calming colors such as blue or green tend to help people relax and slow down.

> › **KEEP BREATHING.** Many people subconsciously hold their breath when holding a strength training posture, as if the breath holding will somehow make the effort seem easier. It doesn't. It makes it harder. Breathe in through your nose and out through your mouth. Whenever you feel as if you can't hold any longer, bring your focus to your breathing and make sure you are doing it!

> › **LISTEN TO CLASSICAL MUSIC.** Music improves the exercise experience. When study participants listen to music, they tend to work out longer and more intensely and feel less fatigued or stressed during their workouts. I've tried many different types of music at my gyms and I've found that classical music serves as the best backdrop for strength training. Pop, rock, and rap music may all work great for cardio, but the beat is just too fast for my

90-Second Sets. If you listen to these types of music, you'll find yourself moving to a fast cadence. You'll be skipping your stopping points and you'll rush through the routine. Even if you don't think you like classical, try it. In the past six years, I've been playing it exclusively and haven't heard a single person complain. I'm only asking you to listen to it for a few minutes before your workout to get you in the right frame of mind and during your workouts to keep you there.

CLASSICAL ALBUMS TO TRY

Great Haydn Symphonies

Mendelssohn: String Symphonies Volume 3

Handel: *Water Music*

> **BE BEAUTIFUL.** It may be true that most people exercise in their basements, but that doesn't make it right. I'll remind you again. You only need a wall and a floor. Every room in your home probably features those two essentials, so do your routine in the most beautiful room in the house. Experiment with locations. One day, try the routine in the most brightly lit room in the house. Another time, try it in front of the TV. Still another time, do it while looking out your largest window.

Once you find your ideal space, decorate it with beautiful artwork. Choose a decor that is serene and beautiful. Choose landscapes, still lifes, or portraits, but stay away from pictures of hard bodies. I don't know many women who feel motivated to do a Wall Sit when they see a picture of Jennifer Aniston or Jennifer Lopez.

LEVEL 1 AT HOME

I know it's hard to believe that two simple movements—movements that, in fact, require no movement whatsoever—could do anything good for your body in such a short period of time, but they do. I'm confident that three minutes is a lot longer than you think! If you are doing no other exercise, I recommend you do the Level 1 routine five times a week, for a total of fifteen weekly minutes. If you do any type of regular cardio, practice yoga, or another form of exercise, do it three times a week (doing your other exercise on your off days). If you are the type of person who needs to exercise every day in order to form that fitness habit, do half of it every day. Do the Wall Sit on a Monday and the Plank on a Tuesday and then the Wall Sit on a Wednesday and the Plank on a Thursday and so on, switching back and forth between the two essential movements each day.

Hold each exercise up to 90 seconds. Time yourself the first time, to see how long you can hold. Most beginners last somewhere between twenty and thirty seconds. Congratulate yourself for your effort and progress from there. Every second is progress. I've changed the rules for you so you can always progress and get closer to your goal.

HOME LEVEL 1 SCORECARD

Copy this chart and use it to track your progress or write it down in a notebook.

MOVEMENT	TIME IN SECONDS
1. Wall Sit	
2. Plank	

PLANK

Arms, chest, abdominals, back, legs, glutes, calves, toes, hands, wrists, neck
(nearly everything except your earlobes)

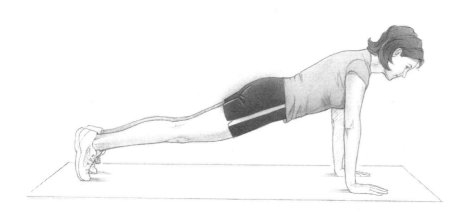

When you get into a Plank position (as shown) every passing second makes muscles weaken. As each muscle becomes more exhausted, other muscles have to get involved to keep the position. Can you do a Plank without your feet? No. So the muscles in your feet, shins, and calves must be doing something. If your glutes and abs aren't contracting, you will sag to the floor. If your shoulder blades aren't contracting to support your chest, shoulders, and triceps, you will plummet to the ground. The wrists hold up the arms and the neck holds up the head. The Plank works your entire beautiful body!

Kneel on your hands and knees. Extend your legs and come into the Plank position by reaching back through your heels and forward through the crown of your head. Keep your shoulders relaxed and low, away from your ears, and keep your hips up. Don't allow your low back to cave downward. Hold, with your arms extended, up to 90 seconds. Don't forget to breathe.

WALL SIT

Legs, butt, abdominals, lower back

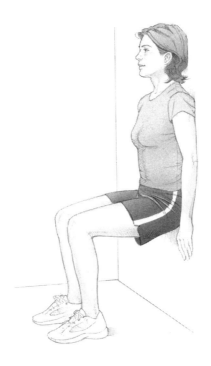

Yes, the Wall Sit works your legs, as you'll soon find out, but it also firms your abs and back as you press your back into the wall. Again, no moving is necessary; just sit still. Press your back against a wall. Walk your feet away from the wall and then slide your back down the wall until your knees form ninety-degree angles. Hold up to ninety seconds. Again, remember to breathe.

That's it. You're done. Go shopping. Meet a friend. Get back to work. Get on with your life.

LEVEL 2 AT HOME

When should you move from Level 1 to Level 2? When you want to. If you'd like, you can stay at Level 1 for the rest of your life. Those two movements strengthen every muscle in your body. Do them regularly and you'll keep those muscles strong and firm.

LEVEL 2 PREREQUISITES

You can hold the Wall Sit for 90 seconds.

You can hold the Plank for 90 seconds.

Move on to Level 2 only when you want more. You might not be able to imagine that you'd ever want to exercise longer and harder. Believe me, you will. It happens to everyone. Fitness and strength build a kind of confidence that is empowering and contagious. Once you feel stronger, you'll want to get even stronger still, and when that happens, it's time for Level 2.

Complete the Level 2 routine three days a week if you are doing no other type of exercise. Do it twice a week if you are doing some cardio, such as walking or cycling.

HOME LEVEL 2 SCORECARD

Copy this chart and use it to track your progress or write it down in a notebook. Do them in this order:

MOVEMENT	TIME IN SECONDS
1. Superwoman	
2. Wall Sit	
3. Leg Raise	
4. Sit-up	
5. Hangin' Out	
6. Plank	

SUPERWOMAN

Upper and lower back, shoulders, neck, glutes, hamstrings

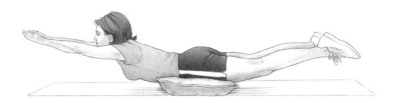

Lie facedown on the floor. Place a thick pillow beneath your hips. Stretch your arms overhead and extend your legs. Raise your arms, head, and legs off the floor. Hold up to 90 seconds. You're flyin' now.

WALL SIT

Legs, butt, abdominals, lower back

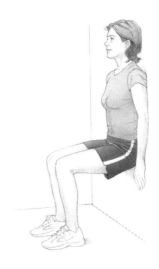

You know what to do. Put your back against the wall, sit, and hold.

LEG RAISE

Abdominals and thighs

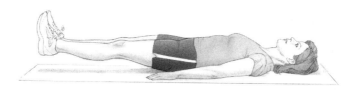

Lie on your back, hands by your sides and with your legs extended. With your legs straight, raise your feet six to eight inches off the floor. Hold for up to 90 seconds.

SIT-UP

Abdominals and thighs

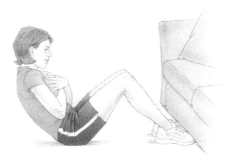

Sit on the floor with your legs bent. Anchor your feet under a couch. Put a pillow under your bottom if you are sitting on a hard surface. Start at the top of a sit-up position and slowly recline back until your body is at a forty-five-degree angle with the floor. Hold for up to 90 seconds.

HANGIN' OUT

Shoulders, back, abdominals, arms, thighs

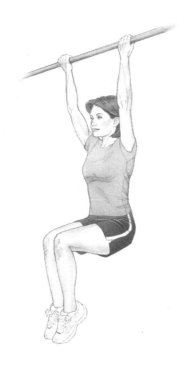

Hangin' Out is the only home exercise that requires a piece of equipment: a chin-up bar. You can find many to choose from in every price range at any sporting goods store.

Do you wonder: How can hanging get me stronger? I'm not even doing anything. Indeed, you are. Hanging is one of the first strength-building exercises Olympic gymnastic centers recommend to young (age two to four) gymnasts who are trying to build the strength to pull themselves up on the uneven bars. If it works for them, it will work for you! Eventually, if you continually work at it, you'll be able to pull yourself all the way up.

Grasp the bar with an underhand grip. Lift your knees until your thighs are parallel with the floor. Lift your body one inch. Hang for up to 90 seconds. Most beginners last somewhere between ten and twenty seconds on the first try. No matter how long you hang for the first time, give yourself a pat on the back and progress from there. If calluses are a concern, buy a pair of workout gloves. This exercise can be done at the playground on the monkey bars if you don't want to invest in a chinning bar.

PLANK

Arms, chest, abdominals, back, legs, glutes, calves, toes, hands, wrists, neck

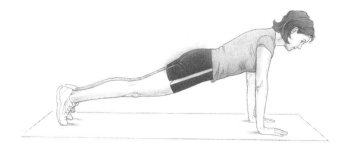

Go ahead, grab some floor.

Great job! You've completed the Level 2 routine. You're done!

LEVEL 3 AT HOME

My advice for moving up to Level 3 is the same as it was for Level 2. Move up when you are ready and willing. Once you can last for 90 seconds on all of the Level 2 movements, and once you feel you want and crave more, then you're ready for Level 3. If you get to 90 seconds on any of the Level 3 exercises, consider yourself a true athlete! Do your Level 3 routine no more than twice a week. If you do cardio on the side, such as Pilates, yoga, walking, running, and cycling, at least twice a week, do this routine just once.

For various exercises, you'll see that I suggest a stop-and-hold technique. Rather than pushing fluidly through a repetition, you'll stop at nine distinct points. This stop-and-hold technique allows you to maximize the hardest part of the movement, getting more out of the exercise in less time.

HOME LEVEL 3 SCORECARD

Copy this chart and use it to track your progress or write it down in a notebook.

MOVEMENT	TIME IN SECONDS
1. Superwoman	
2. Wall Sit	
3. Hindu Squat	
4. Leg Raise	
5. Sit-up	
6. Reverse Pull-up	
7. Push-up	

SUPERWOMAN

Upper and lower back, shoulders, neck, glutes, hamstrings

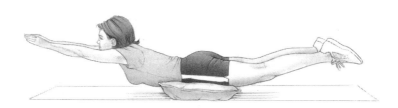

You know what to do. It's time for your liftoff. Hold up to 90 seconds. Focus on your breathing as you hold.

WALL SIT

Legs, butt, abdominals, lower back

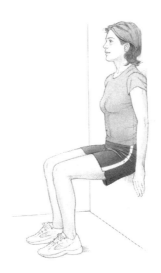

You know what to do. Put your back against the wall, sit, and hold.

HINDU SQUAT

Legs, butt

Stand with your feet a shoulder width apart or a little wider. Raise your arms to shoulder height in front of you for balance. Start the stopwatch, bend your knees, and slowly descend. The first third of the movement is useless, so we want to work the most effective parts of each exercise. Here's where I want you to stop and hold.

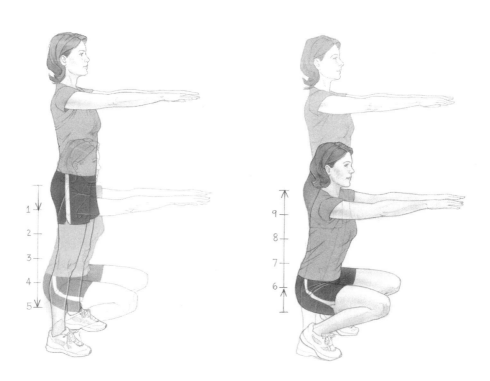

1. When you get about a third of the way down, you will feel your thighs begin to work. Hold for a count of ten seconds.
2. Descend two inches farther, raising your heels as needed, and balancing yourself on the balls of your feet. Use your extended arms for balance, leaning forward slightly as needed.
3. Descend two inches farther.
4. Descend two inches farther.
5. Now you are at the bottom. It's time to start back up. Even though your legs are shaking and burning, maintain form and resist the temptation to come up quickly.
6. Rise two inches and stop and hold for ten seconds.
7. Rise two inches and stop and hold for ten.
8. Rise two inches and stop and hold for ten.
9. Now you're two-thirds of the way up. Hold for ten and then slowly rise to the standing position. Isn't it amazing how one rep feels as if you did the work of 90 or more! In my routine, every second is like doing a rep—so 90 seconds is like doing 90 reps more effectively and without the pump! That's why every second counts!

LEG RAISE

Abdominals

Lie on your back with your legs raised, perpendicular to your torso. Lower your legs slowly toward the floor, stopping when your heels are about two inches away from the floor. Ground your lower back into the floor and tense your abs.

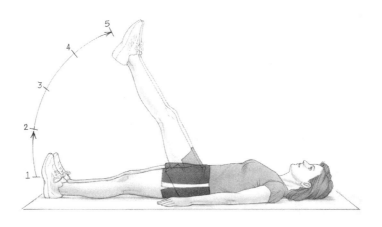

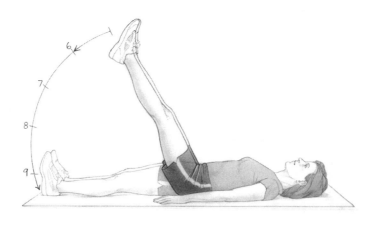

1. You've reached hold number one. Hold here for ten seconds.

2. Raise your feet two inches and hold for ten.

3. Raise your feet two inches and hold for ten.

4. Raise your feet two inches and hold for ten.

5. Now you're about three-quarters of the way up. Hold for ten. It's time to reverse the movement.

6. Drop your feet two inches and hold for ten.

7. Drop your feet two inches and hold for ten.

8. Drop your feet two inches and hold for ten.

9. Now you're two inches from the floor. Hang on for dear life or for ten seconds, whichever you reach first.

SIT-UP

Abdominals

Sit upright with your knees bent. Anchor your feet under the bottom of a couch. Tuck your chin to your chest, round your lower back, and curl your tailbone. Lower just enough to feel your abs contract. This is your first hold.

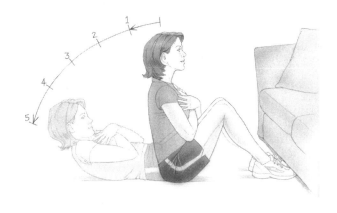

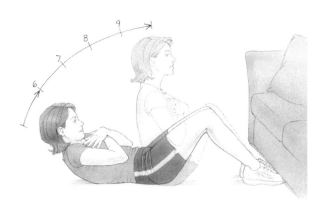

1. Hold for ten.
2. Lower two inches, rounding your back as you lower, and hold for ten.
3. Lower two inches and hold for ten.
4. Lower two inches and hold for ten.
5. Now your lower back is resting on the floor. Don't allow your shoulder blades to touch. Hold for ten. Now we're coming up.
6. Rise two inches and hold for ten.
7. Rise two inches and hold for ten.
8. Rise two inches and hold for ten.
9. You're at your last hold. Your back is flat, but you are leaning back, feeling a good amount of tension in your abs. Hang on. You're almost there. Hold for ten.

REVERSE PULL-UP

Shoulders, arms, upper back, abdominals

Think you can't do a pull-up? Think again. I've taught women with the skinniest of arms to do pull-ups. This isn't just for the GI Janes. You really can do this.

There's nothing like the sense of satisfaction and confidence from completing your first ever pull-up. If you are unable to do a pull-up at this time, try this approach.

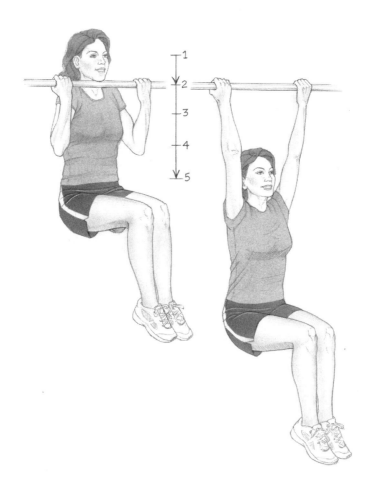

Work at lowering part of the way only until you get strong enough to pull yourself up. Approach your pull-up bar and get yourself to the top position by climbing or boosting yourself up. You will be using an underhand grip, bending your elbows, and bringing your chin over the bar. This is your first hold. Breathing hard already? I bet you are, but you can hang on. Do the best you can.

1. Hold up to ten seconds.
2. Lower two inches and hold up to ten seconds.
3. Lower two inches and hold up to ten seconds.
4. Lower two inches and hold up to ten seconds.
5. Now your arms are outstretched. Pull with your hands, even though your body may not move upward, and hold as much as twenty seconds for a total of sixty seconds. You're done! Great job.

When you are able to do the lowering phase for a total of sixty seconds, take a day or two of rest and then try to do a pull-up from the hanging position. I bet you can do it now! Don't forget to e-mail me when you are able to do your first pull-up. It means a lot to me that you are this successful!

PUSH-UP

Arms, chest, abdominals

You already know how to do the Plank, thanks to your hard efforts during Level 1. Now let's add some movement to that exercise.

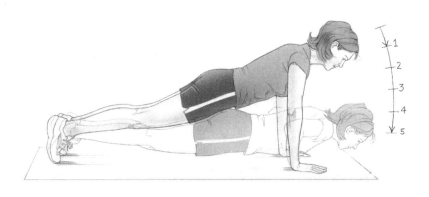

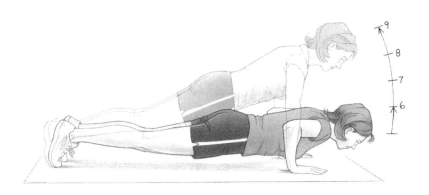

1. Start in the Plank position. Lower yourself two inches and hold for ten.

2. Lower yourself two more inches and hold for ten.

3. Lower yourself two more inches and hold for ten.

4. Lower yourself two more inches and hold for ten.

5. Lower yourself two more inches and hold for ten. Your chest should be two to four inches from the floor. (At this point, people usually accuse me of being a masochist! I'm sure they're kidding.) Keep your hips aligned with your back and remember to breathe!

6. Next, push up two inches and hold for ten seconds.

7. Push up two more inches and hold for ten seconds.

8. Push up two inches higher and hold for ten seconds.

9. Now your arms are fully extended in the plank position. Hold for ten.

Note: If you do the ten-count holds on the way down and can't push back up—don't worry. Most people can't at first. Just do the lowering phase (holds 1 through 5). One day you'll find that you have the strength to come back up. On that day, just get to the top. Don't even attempt to do holds 6 through 9. During your next workout, try hold 6 but skip holds 7 through 9. Then, in a subsequent workout, add another hold. Continue to do so until you're doing all nine holds for a total of one 90-Second Set. Remember— it's all good—there is no failure here. If you are able to increase your time by even *one* second, you win. You are stronger and better.

GET STRONGER AT THE GYM

Let me get something straight right now. You do not have to exercise at the gym. My home routines are short on time and use minimal equipment, but they are wickedly effective. There's no need to force yourself to exercise at a gym if something about the experience makes you apprehensive. I believe in stress-free movement. I don't believe in putting yourself through emotional anguish in order to create a firm, lean body.

That said, keep in touch with these feelings. Many women change their minds about how they feel about the gym as they get stronger. Whereas they may feel intimidated walking into a gym in the beginning, they eventually get strong enough at home that their attitude changes.

When are you ready to try the gym? If you agree with any of the following statements, you're ready:

> You feel as if you could knock out the person behind the desk.

> You like to work out away from home. Gym time is that oasis of downtime in your day when no one—not your boss, your kids, your parents, or your significant other—can pester you with questions, tasks, or informational overload.

> You are interested in taking your strength to a new level, in seeing just how strong and fit you can get. Maybe, like my coauthor, you're the type of person who *likes* to sweat, continually grow stronger, and have muscular guys stare at you in disbelief when you lift three-quarters of a weight stack when they can only do half.

Do my gym routine twice a week if this is your only exercise. If you have other exercise interests—yoga, Pilates, cardio—you can drop back to just once a week. If you really love exercise (you know who you are), you can strength-train as often as twice a week and still do other forms of exercise, but you must pay careful attention to how you schedule your sessions. Schedule as many days between your strength training sessions as possible. For instance, if you strength-train on a Monday, your next session should not be until Thursday. If you do it on a Tuesday, your second session should be Friday. Then do your favorite types of cardio and other types of exercise on your non–strength training days. Keep in mind that strenuous weight-bearing exercise such as running will beat up your body, requiring you to take more off days. If you experience what I like to call Seven Dwarf Syndrome—you're grumpy, sneezy, sleepy, dopey, bashful, and so achy that you need the constant care of Doc—you're overdoing it.

Use the following as a guide.

MONDAY	Weights
TUESDAY	Yoga
WEDNESDAY	Elliptical
THURSDAY	Weights
FRIDAY	Pilates
SATURDAY	Stretch
SUNDAY	Rest

HOW TO CHOOSE A GYM

I have very specialized expensive equipment by the brand MedX at my gym that allows people to lift phenomenal amounts of weight. I'm talking about tiny women doing 200 pounds on the lower-back machine, 600 pounds on the leg press, 200 pounds on the lat pull-down machine, and 160 pounds on the shoulder press. The vast majority of facilities do not have this specialized equipment. If you can find MedX, great. If not, don't worry about it. You can still get a great workout. It just means you won't be able to move as much weight and that you will need to take extra care to set up your machine correctly.

Use these pointers:

> Walk the circuit to see whether the gym has the equipment you need to do the recommended exercises. Most will.

> Notice how you feel when you walk into the gym. Go with your gut. If you feel relaxed and calm, this is the right place for you to exercise. If you feel ashamed, embarrassed, or uptight, it's not.

BEFORE YOU START

To determine how much weight you should initially use, make your first couple of trips to the gym an experimental expedition. For each exercise, do ten reps with a light weight. Move slowly and smoothly. Use control and don't forget to breathe. After your first set, rest. Then add weight and do another set of ten. Continue to add weight until your set feels difficult but not impossible. That's your starting weight. Write it down on your scorecard (see page 62) and progress to the next exercise.

Take two or three days off. Return to the gym. Use the weights that you wrote down and do ten slow reps. If you feel you can lift more, add weight and do a second set. Again, your goal is to do a difficult but not impossible set of ten. Is that all you can do without sacrificing your form? Then that's your starting weight or "working" weight for the routines to follow. Make a note of it.

Do this test every six months to see your progress.

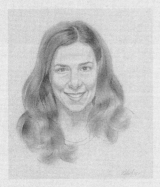

JULIE SIEGEL

When I turned forty, I realized I was not as firm as I would have liked to be. I had put on weight during the winter. Usually I'm able to get it back off in the spring just by walking more as the weather gets warmer. Last year was different. The weight didn't come off as it had in the past.

I realized I probably needed a formal exercise approach, but I have three kids and I work in Manhattan four days a week. I'm gone twelve hours on my workdays. I don't have a lot of free time to spend at the gym.

I started training with Pete about nine months ago. He eased me into it and made it progressively more difficult over time. In just six weeks I saw changes in my body. My clothes fit differently. I'd bought new pants, and they fit better than my older pants. In the past nine months, I've dropped a full clothing size, from a six to a four, and I lost ten pounds on the scale. I'm more toned, and I can now eat more without gaining weight.

YOUR GYM OPTIONS

I choose the seven exercises shown on pages 64 to 71 because they are the most effective exercises you can do at the gym. They are big exercises that work multiple muscle groups at once. They are also the easiest machines to set up, and the most user-friendly in terms of using proper form and technique. Learn and master this one set of exercises and stick with it. What changes is *how* you do the exercises. In the following pages, you'll find three movement options to keep you mentally stimulated. Feel free to mix and match Options 1, 2, and 3. Go with the flow. In the same session, you might stick with just one option or you might alternate between two or all three of them.

OPTION 1
THREE REPS IN 90 SECONDS
AKA
3/90

Picture a very athletic and capable person. Let's make this specific: picture Arnold Schwarzenegger. Now picture me training him. He's a strong guy, right? Think he can do a lot of push-ups? Let's see. I tell him to get down on the floor and do ninety push-ups in 90 seconds. Can you picture how fast he'd be pumping out those push-ups? Next I ask Arnold to do twelve reps in 90 seconds. Doesn't that paint a different picture? More control? Smoother reps? Finally I tell him to do just three reps in 90 seconds. Can you picture the effort and control that goes into those three reps? It sounds difficult, doesn't it? That's our game, 3/90. Your goal is to do as few reps as possible in 90 seconds, with the ultimate goal being three.

Start by timing yourself and see how many reps you do in 90 seconds. The first time you do this, lift normally, count, and watch the clock. Write down the number of reps on your scorecard and then try to do fewer reps in 90 with each successive workout.

Keep in mind that some exercises are better suited for fewer reps than others. For example, it's easier to do a shoulder press, with its long range of motion, in three reps than the leg abduction machine, which has a much shorter range of motion. For leg abduction, you'll probably only be able to get yourself down to six to eight reps in 90 seconds. To know when it's time to increase the weight, use this guide:

> For big exercises that work multiple muscle groups (lower back machine, leg press, row, shoulder press): increase the weight once you can do three or fewer reps in 90 seconds.

> For small exercises that zero in on one muscle group (abdominal machine, rotary torso machine, leg abduction machine): increase the weight once you can do six or fewer reps.

OPTION 2
90-SECOND REPS WITH STEPS
AKA
STEP/90

You can use Option 1 as long as you wish. Options 2 and 3 are here for you when you need variety. You'll know you need it when it happens. One day, you'll walk into the gym and you'll say to yourself, I don't feel like doing 3/90 today. When that happens, you're ready for Option 2 or 3. For Option 2, you increase the mental and physical challenge by doing one rep with holds or "steps." Move the weight about two inches at a time and hold each position for ten seconds each time. Divide the rep into nine parts. For details on precisely where to stop and hold for each exercise, consult the numbers that accompany the exercise illustrations on pages 64 to 71. Each number counts as one of your steps.

OPTION 3
INCREMENTALLY INCREASE THE WEIGHT
AKA
LADDER/90

I call Option 3 the Ladder because the method resembles the motion of climbing and descending a ladder, but in this case the ladder is your weight stack. Start with a medium weight, about 30 to 40 percent lighter than the heaviest weight you can lift. Lift or push the weight out an inch and hold for ten seconds. Then complete the rep. Add ten to twenty pounds and do it again. Continue to climb up the weight stack a total of five steps, adding more weight each time. Then descend four steps for 90 seconds of total work. Was the last step easy to hold? Then start ten pounds heavier next time.

GYM SCORECARD

Copy this chart and use it to track your progress
or write it down in a notebook.

Movement	WEIGHT	TIME	REPS	OPTION	NOTES
Abduction machine					
Lower-back machine					
Leg press					
Rotary torso machine					
Abdominal machine					
Row					
Shoulder press					

THE ROUTINE

In the following routine, I tried to choose machines that are available at most gyms. If you can't find a machine, you can either skip that movement or you can substitute a similar exercise. Use this advice:

DO THE EXERCISES IN THE ORDER LISTED. I have developed this order over the years to give you fast results.

KEEP BREATHING. Many people hold their breath when they lift, but this is counter-productive and may even be dangerous. Research completed at Loma Linda University in California has determined that average blood pressure during heavy lifting soared to 311/284 when study participants held their breath. On the other hand, when they slowly exhaled as they pressed the weight, blood pressure only increased to an average (and safe) 198/174. Breathing into the lift will also help you to relax and concentrate your mental effort on lifting the weight. I think you'll find that you not only enjoy your workout more when you breathe slowly, deeply, and regularly but also be able to push more weight. If you can't breathe slowly, breathe fast (like Lamaze breathing).

LISTEN TO CLASSICAL MUSIC. Most gyms play hard rock, club music, or something loud and fast. Load up some classical music albums on your MP3 player or CD player and listen to them through headphones.

IGNORE THE INQUIRING MINDS. Most people at the gym only know one way to lift. They pump out a bunch of reps. They rest, and then they do it again. It pains me to watch this. It's like sticking a bunch of people in a round room and telling them to find the corner! Even though you may be the only person at your gym who is moving the weight so slowly—and, gasp, holding the weight in one position for as long as ten seconds—*you're* the one who is getting results. People will stare at you. Some may actually ask you why you are lifting it that way. You can almost rest assured that some bodybuilder will eventually approach you and offer to show you the "right" way to do it. While she was lifting at the YMCA one day and holding a weight for ten seconds, my coauthor, Alisa, was approached by a fitness instructor who asked, "Are you okay?" She said that she was, and the instructor asked, "You're holding the weight *on purpose?*" The instructor walked away, shaking her head.

Don't let it get to you. You'll prove them all wrong when you transform your body. How can anyone argue with your firm arms and legs? They can't, and if they ask you a second time, tell them to call me. I'll take care of it.

1. ABDUCTION MACHINE

Outer thighs

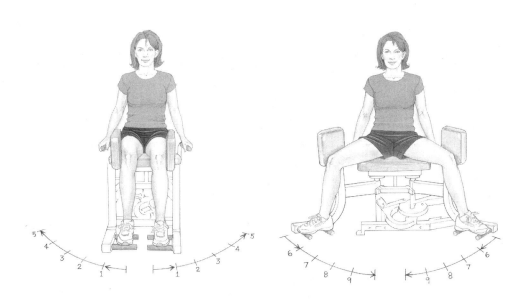

Sit in the machine with your legs inside the pads.

Option 1: Slowly push your knees apart as far as they will go and then slowly return to the starting position. Repeat, aiming for as few reps as possible in 90 seconds.

Option 2: Stop for ten seconds at each of the nine steps shown on the accompanying illustration.

Option 3: Push your knees apart to Position 5, hold for ten, slowly return to the start, and climb and descend your ladder, as described on page 61.

2. LOWER-BACK MACHINE

Lower back, thighs, butt

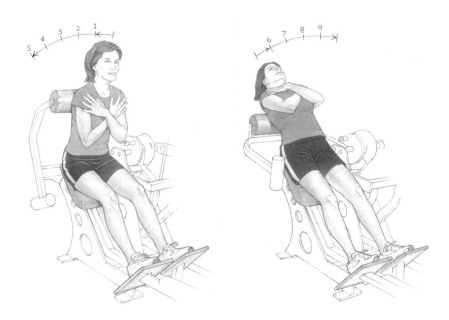

Adjust the machine so that the pads are just behind your shoulder blades. Attach the seat belt. You're going to need it. Sit up tall. Arch your back. Cross your arms over your chest.

Option 1: Slowly lean back as far as you can. Don't worry if your bottom lifts off the seat a little. This only makes the exercise even more effective, working your back, butt, and legs. Slowly return to the start and repeat, aiming for as few reps as possible in 90 seconds.

Option 2: Stop for ten seconds at each of the nine steps shown on the accompanying illustration.

Option 3: Lean back four to six inches to Position 2. You will be sitting upright. Hold for ten, finish the rep, release, and climb and descend your ladder.

3. LEG PRESS

Thighs, butt, abdominals, back

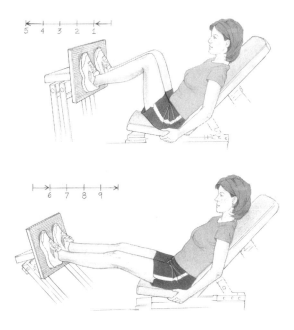

Sit in the leg-press machine. Place your feet on the platform, spacing them a shoulder's distance apart. Adjust the machine so that your legs are bent at a ninety-degree angle and so that you are sitting up rather than reclining. Place the seat back between fifty-five and seventy-five degrees. This requires your body to use more muscles, making the exercise more effective.

Option 1: Slowly press the platform away from you as you extend your legs. Then slowly return to the start. Repeat, aiming for as few reps as possible in 90 seconds.

Option 2: Stop for ten seconds at each of the nine steps shown on the accompanying illustration.

Option 3: Push the platform two inches to Position 1 and hold for ten seconds. Finish the rep, release, and then climb and descend your ladder.

4. ROTARY TORSO MACHINE

Waist, abdominals, back

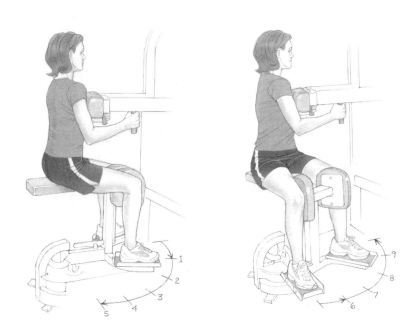

Sit in the machine and adjust it to fit you according to the manufacturer's instructions. All machines will have a sign attached to tell you how to set it up.

Option 1: Twist to your right as far as you can go, keeping your spine extended. Return to the start and repeat, aiming for a total of three reps in 90 seconds. Then adjust the machine to go in the reverse direction.

Option 2: Stop for ten seconds at each of the steps shown on the accompanying illustration.

Option 3: Twist two inches to Position 1 and hold for ten seconds, finish the rep, release, and then climb and descend your ladder. Repeat on the other side.

5. ABDOMINAL MACHINE

Abdominals

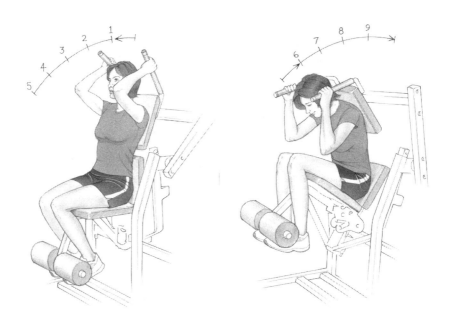

Your gym may have one of two types of abdominal machines (or possibly both). In one type, you sit on a seat and exercise your abdomen by pushing forward against a pad that fits across your chest. In another type, you sit but work your abs by simultaneously pulling forward and down on handles with your hands and forward and up against another set of levers with your ankles. This is the type I've chosen to depict in the accompanying illustration, but feel free to use whatever machine your gym offers. If your gym offers a few types, try them all and see which type you like best. If you like them all, alternate among them for variety.

The following will work for either type of seated abdominal machine. Adjust the machine according to the manufacture's instructions.

Option 1: Pull forward slowly as far as you can go, then slowly return to the start. Repeat, aiming for as few reps as possible in 90 seconds.

Option 2: Stop for ten seconds at each of the numbered steps shown on the accompanying illustrations.

Option 3: Push forward two inches to Position 1 and hold for ten seconds. Finish the rep, return to the start, and then climb and descend your ladder.

6. ROW

Upper back, shoulders, biceps

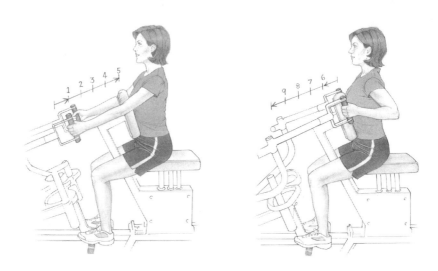

Most gyms have two types of rowing machines. With one, you sit on a seat, press your chest into a stationary pad, grasp a pair of handlebars, and pull them toward you. For the other, you sit on a platform with your legs extended, grab a bar attached to a cable, and pull it toward you. Try both and see which one you relate to. They both work effectively. Whichever type you use, grasp the handles with a neutral grip and pull toward you. Keep your shoulders low, back flat, and head and neck relaxed.

Option 1: Slowly pull the handles or cable toward your upper abdomen, keeping your shoulders low. Bring your elbows as far back as you can. Return to the starting position. Repeat, aiming for as few reps as possible in 90 seconds.

Option 2: Stop for ten seconds at each of the numbered steps shown on the accompanying illustration.

Option 3: Pull to Position 5 on the accompanying illustration. Your elbows should be as far back as you can get them and the bar or handles as close to your torso as you can get them. Hold for ten seconds. Return to the start and then climb and descend your ladder.

7. SHOULDER PRESS

Shoulders, trapezius, neck, triceps

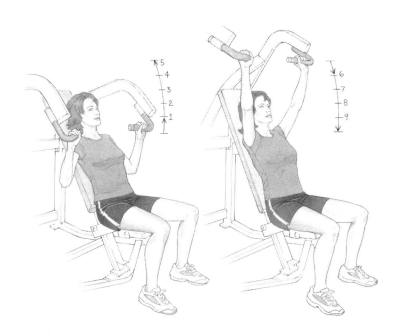

Sit in the machine and adjust the handles to shoulder height.

Option 1: Slowly press the handles upward, extending your arms. Once your arms are almost fully extended, slowly lower to the starting position. Repeat, aiming for as few reps as possible in 90 seconds.

Option 2: Stop for ten seconds at each of the numbered steps shown on the accompanying illustrations.

Option 3: Press the handles up to Position 3 and hold for ten seconds. Finish the rep, return to the start, and then climb and descend your ladder.

THE WONDER WOMAN
WORKOUT

Let me clear up any anxiety you might feel as you read this section. You are not required to do this workout if you are not up to it! Any home workout level and any gym option will get you incredibly fit, sexy, and confident. If you are pressed for time, you do not need to add more.

So why do I have a Wonder Woman Workout at all? Because I've met a few women who, once they start working out with the 90-Second method, get addicted. They can't stop. They beg me for more. They want to see just how strong they can get. They want a challenge. They want to push their limits.

Take my coauthor, Alisa. When we met, she told me that she had tried strength training off and on. Staying "on" required a great deal of mental discipline for her, as she hated it. She loved other forms of exercise, such as running, but she hated the weight room. She wanted stronger bones, firmer muscles, and a tighter body, but she didn't want to spend an hour in the gym a few times a week to get them.

I suggested she start with the Plank and Wall Sit. She did. Soon she was calling me, asking, "Shouldn't I be doing more?" I told her, "No, just do what you are doing." She wouldn't leave me alone, though. She loved how her body was changing. Her arms and shoulders were firm. Her legs were strong. She was able, for the first time ever, to lift the big water jugs and place them in the watercooler.

She kept asking for more, so I gave it to her. Soon she was doing the push-up with steps and Hangin' Out. Then I had her add the sit-up. Then she progressed to a full pull-up. Then she joined a gym. She started with the basic set of movements that I recommended but continued to add to them. She added machines. She finished off each workout by seeing how long she could hold a Wall Sit or Plank.

She told me she felt more confident than ever. She loved how the muscular bodybuilders stared at her in disbelief as she held a Plank with her feet balanced on a fitness ball for 90 seconds. She felt like Wonder Woman and wanted other women to know that feeling. She talked me into creating and adding the following challenging movements to the book.

If you are an Alisa, then the following movements are for you. Do them at the end of your gym or home session. See how long you can hold one or more of the following moves. Keep track of your seconds. Consider your seconds your score, and each time you do the routine, see if you can increase your score.

WALL SIT

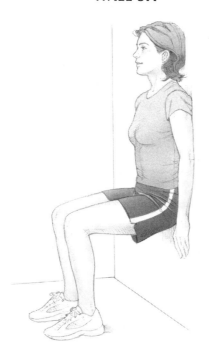

Sit as long as you can. Three minutes is a great initial goal. *Tip:* Do the wall sit while you watch television. The television will distract you, helping you to hold longer than usual.

X PLANK

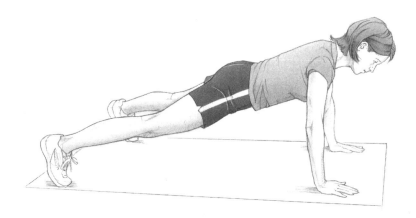

Similar to the Plank, the X Plank ups the ante by spreading your hands and feet in a wider stance. Place your hands on the floor six inches wider than your shoulders and your feet as wide as you can. Now hold. You'll start shaking within seconds. Three minutes is a great initial goal.

HANGIN' OUT

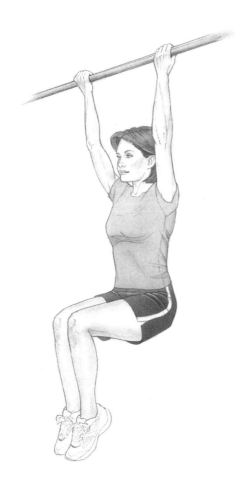

Again, you are looking to break a record. Hang as long as you can.

Don't be afraid to mix and match. Remember, it all works. You can also challenge yourself with the following tips:

> Try the Wall Sit with your baby or toddler in your lap. It will add resistance—making the exercise more effective—and keep your child entertained while you get in your workout. Give your toddler the watch or countdown timer to hold as you both keep track of the time together.

> Add resistance to the Wall Sit by placing a pile of books in your lap or holding dumbbells in your hands.

> Do the Plank with a small child on your back, holding up to 90 seconds.

> Do the push-up with a small child on your back.

> Do the push-up, but hold Point 9 as long as you can.

> Do the Plank with your thighs, shins, or feet on a fitness ball.

> Try to accomplish physical fitness tests that frustrated you as a child. Do you have access to a gym with a knotted rope? Try climbing it. Do you frequent playgrounds with your children? See if you can tame the monkey bars.

HELP FOR SPECIAL BODIES

I want you to push yourself during your 90-Second workouts, but there are also times when I want you to ease up. They include:

> **ILLNESS.** If you have or are recovering from a bout of the flu or any other illness that leaves you physically exhausted, your body needs rest. Now is not the time to lift the heaviest weights you can.

> › **INJURY.** If you have a torn hamstring, sore back, or injured shoulder, you don't want to go heavy on the trouble zone. Go heavy for the movements that don't affect your injury, but ease up on the trouble zone until it heals.

In both cases, I want you to go light, doing what I call PT/90, with PT standing for physical therapy. Do the exercises I prescribe for 90 seconds each with light weight, aiming for six to twelve reps per set. You want to do light weights to get the blood moving and work the range of motion. In the following pages you'll find specific movements to do or add for specific injuries.

BAD KNEES

I train many people who tell me they don't want to work their legs with the Wall Sit or the Leg Press because they have bad knees. In many cases they can actually do these exercises without inflaming their knees, but they are too fearful to try. To reduce the fear, I suggest a simple movement that I call the Magic Knee. It's really simple. You sit at the end of the chair and raise one leg until it is parallel to the floor and hold for sixty seconds. Lower that leg, then raise the other leg.

Because it requires no equipment and no movement, it generates no fear. I'm willing to put money on the fact that you are willing to try the Magic Knee, even though you may not be willing to try the Wall Sit just yet. That's fine. In fact, go ahead and do it. Since you're reading this book, you're already sitting down. Stick a leg out, hold, and see what happens.

No pain or discomfort, right? That's what I thought. Harder than you expected? Yep, thought you'd say that.

The Magic Knee increases circulation to your legs, which relieves the stiffness and soreness. Many of my knee rehabilitation clients find that they can do the Magic Knee and then follow up with a Wall Sit or leg press. Patricia was one of them. I met her at a party. She is five foot two, 180 pounds, and sixty-six years old. As things normally go for me at parties, various friends commented that they were overweight, out of shape, and that nothing seemed to help. They bemoaned that they had no time for long, involved workouts. I couldn't resist. I told them I wanted to show them something, and I recommended they all do the Wall Sit.

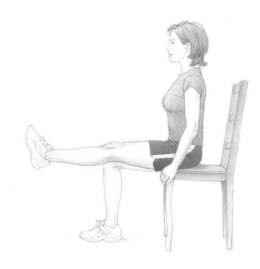

Patricia balked. She refused to try it. When I asked her why, she told me that the pain in her knees was just too much and she was sure that she couldn't sit against the wall or get down on the floor to try a Plank either. I recommended she try the Magic Knee. She tried it and not only did it well but went on to do the Wall Sit and Plank for 90 seconds each! Great job, Patricia. She told me, "My knees haven't felt this good in years."

BAD BACK

If you have a bad back, you can do all of the home routines without irritating it. In fact, Superwoman will make your back stronger and feel better. This is due to the special way I prescribe the exercise. Instead of hyperextending your lower back—a movement some experts say is harmful—I suggest you place a thick pillow under your hips. This allows you to extend without hyperextending.

At the gym avoid using heavy weight on the lower-back machine. Instead use the PT/90 approach on that machine twice a week for a month and then switch to the 3/90 method and crank up the weights. For the Superwoman exercise, raise and hold for ten seconds and repeat nine times for a total of ninety.

SORE SHOULDERS

I see a lot of bad shoulders in my former tennis players, softball players, and golfers. To rehabilitate one or both shoulders I recommend a simple dumbbell overhead press of six to twelve reps in 90 seconds. If you are able to reach over your head all the way, do the Hangin' Out exercise to stretch the shoulder while working your other muscles. At the gym, do use the shoulder-press machine but use the PT/90 technique on that machine. Do not put any weight on, or just use the lightest setting. Move slowly through the fullest range of motion that does not cause pain. Try to increase your range of motion each session. As your shoulder improves, slowly add more weight until you feel more confident and your injury is healed.

Avoid push-ups and the chest press, as both will irritate a shoulder problem.

STRENGTHEN YOUR GOLF SWING

My basic routines will make you a better athlete no matter what your favorite sport. If you run, you'll have more oomph with every stride. If you cycle, you'll have a faster, smoother cadence and climb hills like Lance Armstrong. If you swim, you'll feel less winded after every lap. You do not need to do any additional exercises to strengthen your body for these sports. The basic routines in this chapter are all you need.

If you golf, however, I recommend you do one additional exercise to strengthen your drive and protect your back. If you don't play golf, you can use it to strengthen your abs and define your waistline. Do this exercise especially if you do not have access to a rotary torso machine at the gym.

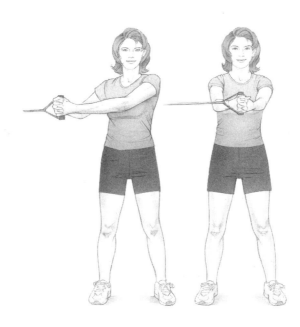

You'll need a set of elastic exercise bands with handles. Wrap the band around a doorknob or other stationary object. Clasp the handles in each hand, your hands together. Stand with your right side toward the door. Extend and raise your arms in front to just below chest height. Step to the right until you create tension in the band. Pull the handles to your left, until you reach the center line of your body. Hold for ten seconds. Relax and repeat eight times for a total of 90 seconds. Then turn and repeat on the other side.

THE SHORTEST CARDIO
AND STRETCHING PLANS EVER

Many women tell me that they hate cardio. "If you hate it, then don't do it," is always my reply, which shocks most of them.

Okay, you're still reading, so that means you must be an exercise lover. Good for you. I've met a few women like you over the years. In fact, my coauthor, Alisa, is addicted to the sensation of having her heart beat faster and sweat dripping down her face. I don't hold it against her, as long as she remembers to take a shower. I tell her, as I'm telling you, that you can do all the cardio you want. I just want to keep you healthy, and by that, I'm talking about your joints.

When it comes to joints—the hips, knees, shoulders, elbows, and other places where one bone meets another—there are two kinds of people. There's the person who can play hard, harder, and hardest and never suffer a day of stiffness or discomfort. Then there are the rest of us. You would think that power walking, tennis, and cycling would be the prescription to a healthy and happy lifestyle, but that's only true if you're built for it. For instance, if I took up running, I would be the proud owner of new knees via knee-replacement surgery within a year or two, and I'm only in my early forties.

My dad is another great example. When I was a child, my hero was (and still is) my dad. He was the biggest, strongest, toughest guy around. Throughout my childhood, he jogged, played tennis, cycled, and lifted weights. In his sixties he entered and made it through the New York City marathon. A few years later he had both hips replaced. At six feet tall and 220 pounds, my dad found his hips couldn't handle all of the grinding. Now in his seventies, his knees are going too.

If you are the type of person who has never experienced knee or any other type of joint pain in your life, then you can probably go ahead and run until you are sixty, seventy, eighty, ninety, or a hundred. You can keep playing tennis, squash, or racquet-

SHEILA HANNA

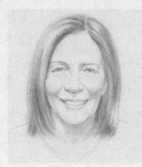

When my gynecologist diagnosed me with osteo-porosis, she told me that I needed to start strength training. I'd already lost an inch in height and I didn't want to lose any more. I'd always walked for fitness and I loved it. Getting up at 6 A.M. to walk six or seven miles was a treat. I thought I was doing the right thing by walking, but my knees hurt terribly, especially when I walked uphill. Yet another doctor, an orthopedist, diagnosed me with osteoarthritis. Just as my gynecologist had, he also recommended strength training.

Two women recommended Pete to me. They were in great shape, and one of them was older than me. I found it hard to believe that one session a week could help me at all, but I decided to give it a try.

The results have been remarkable. My gynecologist had told me that the best I could hope for at my age was to stop the bone loss. Now, with Pete's program and bone-building medication, my bone density is, in my doctor's words, "just shy of normal." I no longer have any pain in my knees. I can easily take hills. I now look better in my clothes too. I'm more toned and I've grown. I remember arguing with my doctor the day she told me I was only five-feet three and a half inches tall. I told her, "No that must be wrong. I'm five-foot four." Now I really am. The strength training has improved my posture and strengthened the bones in my spine, so I've gained back that half inch in height. It also helps me reduce stress. My husband always says that it's a better weekend if I've been to the gym!

Whenever I tell friends about Pete's workout, they say, "Oh that's a scam. That's a rip-off. What makes you think twenty minutes a week could possibly do anything?" As my body changed and my posture improved, however, they started asking, "What are you doing? Are you dieting?" I just said, "No, it's just as I told you. It's this strength training program."

Then they signed up too.

ball too. If you're like me or my dad, however, and you're older than thirty-five, your joints are going to start fighting back. If you feel stiff in the morning and achy after exercise, then I've got bad news. You've got roughly ten thousand miles left in those knees, maybe fewer. Your cartilage is already wearing down. Although you may not be officially diagnosed, I'm willing to bet that you have osteoarthritis. As soon as cartilage starts to wear down, the clock toward needing a joint replacement is ticking. Unlike the clock on your wall, however, you can slow down time by doing the following: not using the joint. The less friction and impact you inflict on the joint, the longer you can go before needing a new one.

It's my goal to get you to your hundredth birthday without having to go under the knife. That's why I have you do so few reps in the strength training program. The less you move and use the joint, the less friction you create and the more cartilage you preserve. Plus my program will build strength in the muscles around your joints, helping to absorb some of the impact from your daily activities. Weight-bearing cardio by nature does not cause osteoarthritis, but it speeds up its progression. If you have any joint discomfort, Pete's orders are this: stop running. If the discomfort is in your shoulder, stop playing racket sports.

This doesn't mean you can't do cardio if you love it. Just switch to nonimpact activities such as swimming, cycling, or even pool running. Yoga is just as good as Pilates, and Pilates is just as good as walking, and walking is just as good as swimming. Do what you enjoy. Go ahead and experiment. Try new things. Keep an open mind. Thinking about that boot camp class at the gym? Try it. Interested in learning how to belly dance? Then do it. Curious about that tai chi class? Take it. Give it a few weeks. If you don't like it, then drop out. And of course, if it doesn't agree with your joints, then just don't do it.

Still, I know you're looking for a specific recommendation from me. You want me to give you a should, and, okay, my editor told me that I had to give you a should too. Here's what I'm going to do. I'll let you choose from the following options. Use these suggestions:

If you love the sensation of feeling "stretched out" and need help with reducing stress: Sign up for a yoga class once or twice a week. Stay away from power yoga and ashtanga styles. You're already getting plenty of strengthening with my plan. Look into more gentle styles of yoga.

If you love having your heart pound but have bad knees: Do my elliptical workout. Warm up for five minutes and then go hard for one minute and easy for one minute. Start with five bursts of faster effort and work your way up to a total of ten bursts, for a total exercise time of twenty minutes. Try to get your heart rate to 80 percent of your max during the faster segments. Then cool down for five minutes at the end.

If your doctor has put the fear of God into you about the need to do more cardio, and you're just not quite sure whether you should trust me over him but you really do hate cardio: Walk. It's easy, it's simple, and you can do it while you are on your way to somewhere else. If you live in a small town or a city, walk as you complete errands, using your own two feet to take you to the post office, the bank, and so on. If you live in suburbia, walk in your neighborhood before or after dinner, take short walking breaks at work, or walk as you window-shop at the mall. Aim for thirty minutes a day.

If you wake stiff in the morning: Do this simple stretching routine to warm up your body to face the day.

> **SPINAL FLEX:** Lie on the floor on your tummy with your elbows bent and palms on the floor. Extend your legs. Press into your hands to lift your torso, arching your back only as much as is comfortable. Keep your hip bones in contact with the floor. It's like doing a push-up with your hips on the floor. Hold for a count of ten, lower, and repeat up to nine times for a total of 90 seconds.

> **ROLL DOWN:** Stand with your feet slightly wider than your hips. Bend your knees slightly. Raise your arms overhead. Tuck in your chin and ex-

hale as you roll down, curling your spine. Reach your hands between your knees as far as you can, bending your knees if needed. Then inhale as you roll back up. When you come to standing position, reach your arms overhead, straighten your spine, and reach laterally to the right as you exhale. Inhale to center. Then bend sideways to the left. Once you come back to center, repeat the entire three-part sequence three times.

Okay, enough stretching. Go get coffee and then turn to chapter 3.

CHAPTER 3

Simplify Your Eating

If you've tried to follow any diet or healthy eating plan over the long term, the math can easily make you feel as if you're back in that high school or college statistics class. Various plans tell you to:

> Balance carbohydrates, fats, and protein in specific ratios, such as 60-20-20 or 40-30-30.

> Count up the number of different colored fruits and vegetables you eat in a day, making sure to consume something red, something purple, something orange, something yellow, and so on.

> Add up salt as you eat it, making sure you do not go over 2,300 daily milligrams.

> Eat equal amounts of omega-3 fatty acids and omega-6 fatty acids.

> Consume two cups of fruit, three cups of dairy, three ounces of whole grains, and two and a half cups of vegetables every day.

To boost mood and energy, strengthen bones, reduce joint discomfort and pain, and improve total body health, follow Pete's Four Simple Rules:

1. Eat Real Food: vegetables, legumes, meat, eggs, nuts and seeds, olive oil, and a limited amount of cheese.
2. Load up on Vegetables and Legumes: include them with every meal.
3. Drink Real Beverages: think water, coffee, and wine!
4. Limit Red Meat: consume it no more than once a week.

You can drop as much as four pounds in three days with the Skinny Black Dress Diet. It involves four steps or phases:

STEP 1: A protein-shake diet for one to three days to drop four pounds.

STEP 2: A protein-shake-avocado-salad diet for two weeks to drop up to six more pounds.

STEP 3: A limited-menu diet to lose up to two pounds a week until you reach your goal.

STEP 4: Follow Pete's Four Simple Rules to maintain your weight loss.

I have a hard time believing that Wilma Flintstone thought about such complicated calculations as she foraged for food. She didn't stumble across a red pepper and say to herself, Oh, I've had a lot of red today. I really need green. I'll leave this here and keep looking. She didn't turn down the wild boar her hairy hubby proudly brought home on his spear, complaining, "Oh honey, you're always bringing home saturated fats. Can't you hunt for some omega-3s instead?"

She didn't, and you shouldn't either. Think about it this way. Our bodies evolved from the Wilma Flintstones of yesteryear. (In my case, I'm a descendent of Fred.) Our bodies learned to use the foods and nutrients that Wilma and Fred ate, and Wilma and

Fred ate simple foods: vegetables, fruit, seeds, nuts, eggs, and meat. When it comes to nutrition, figuring out what and how much to eat should be as simple as asking yourself: What would Wilma eat? I pose that very question repeatedly throughout this chapter.

In the following pages you will find two simple plans to guide your eating. One is designed to get you your healthiest ever, and the other is to help you drop excess pounds. It's my hope that these approaches to eating erase all of your excuses for not eating healthfully!

THE REAL FOOD DIET

You really can eat your way to a longer life and improved well-being, and you can do it in a delicious and simple way. The Real Food Diet will:

> Strengthen your bones.

> Reduce risk for heart disease, cancer, and diabetes.

> Heighten energy.

> Improve sleep.

> Lift your mood.

> Improve memory and concentration.

Perhaps most important, it will add years to your life—years that are so filled with energy, quality, and happiness that you will be ecstatic that you stole them from the Grim Reaper. How do you eat your way to a younger, healthier body? Just follow Pete's Four Simple Rules.

RULE 1:
EAT REAL FOOD

I've put this rule first because it's the most important rule of all. If you can't find the motivation to follow all Four Rules, then at least follow this one. It's *that* important. Researchers from Harvard estimate that 80 percent of heart disease, 70 percent of strokes, and 90 percent of type 2 diabetes could be eliminated if we all ate real foods. A recent study from the National Institutes of Health of more than 380,000 participants determined that people who most closely followed a diet composed of real foods—vegetables, fruit, nuts, fish, meat, and whole grains—were dramatically less likely to die from cancer or heart disease than people who tended to eat fake foods.

What are real foods? That's easy. They look like real foods. Go to the grocery store and see for yourself. If you can figure out where something came from, it's a real food. Lettuce? Yep, it's real food. It came from the ground. An orange? Yep, it's a real food. It came from a tree. Eggs? You got it. They came from a hen. Real foods include the fruit, vegetables, beans, nuts, and seeds that grow in soil, along with the meat, milk, and eggs from animals. Here's another hint that can help you tell the difference between real foods and fake foods. Real foods go bad. They spoil. Keep them for too long, and mold starts to grow on them, they start to stink, and they turn funny colors. (My friends, oddly, say the same about me.) Fake food? Put a Twinkie on your windowsill and let it sit there for a few months. Anything? Nope, still looks, smells, and tastes like a Twinkie, doesn't it? That should tell you something.

Studies consistently show that real foods contain nutrients our bodies need for optimal health. Real foods provide:

> › Antioxidants to protect cells throughout the body from the damaging effects of smog, smoke, ultraviolet light, stress, and food toxins. These

MICHELE KAPLAN

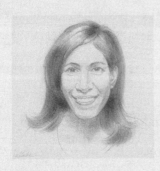

I started training with Pete about six months ago, mostly to lose weight. I'm forty-five, and everything I'd tried before Pete just hadn't worked. I'd use the elliptical at the gym for forty-five minutes to an hour every single day. When I finished that workout, I was starving, and then I would end up eating foods like bagels that I'd been trying not to eat. The long minutes of cardio were getting me nowhere.

When one of my friends saw me in the gym one day, she asked me, "Why are you working out for an hour a day? You don't have to work out this much." She told me about Pete and suggested I give his method a try. I was leery. I'd stayed away from strength training because I didn't want big muscles. I also didn't think I would be strong enough to do it.

Pete's workout was a struggle at first, but I always felt good about going. Now I actually enjoy Pete's workout, and I would like to do it more often!

Pete suggested some dietary changes too, encouraging me to eat more avocados, chicken, and fish and fewer bagels and other flour-based foods. Now I prepare simple dishes. I'll bake a salmon and steam some vegetables or I'll have shrimp cocktail with vegetables. When I'm really in a hurry, perhaps to shuttle my kids to various sporting activities, I have Pete's avocado dinner. It really makes me feel full, and I love the taste. It also seems to help balance my blood sugar.

I now have more energy and I use it to do a lot more walking. I can even run up a flight of stairs without feeling winded. I definitely feel like Pete's workout sped up my metabolism. I also didn't realize how much my lower back was hurting until Pete's workouts stopped the nagging pain. I used to wake up with it stiff, and now I wake up feeling good.

I now feel my abdominal muscles; I never felt muscles there before. I see definition in my arms too. I'm also buying jeans again. I would not have been trying on jeans a year ago, but I've lost about ten pounds and I feel so much more comfortable in them now.

wonder nutrients fend off cancer, heart disease, and wrinkles and probably preserve memory too.

› Vitamins and minerals that our bodies need for cell reactions, stronger bones, and muscle maintenance.

› Fiber to fill us up, normalize blood sugar levels, and keep us regular.

› Important essential fats for brain health, mood, heart health, fertility, and more.

› Protein to help muscles recover and get stronger from your workouts.

I can almost hear your thoughts. If you're not thinking this right about now, you'll think it soon. You'll think about a few real foods—foods like eggs, avocados, and coconuts—and you'll think, Pete, these real foods are loaded with fat. Aren't they bad for me? In a word, no.

Don't worry about the natural fat that comes from real foods. Ask yourself, What would Wilma eat? Would she not eat an egg because she was worried about the fat? Research has shown over and over again that natural sources of fat do not raise your risk for any disease. In fact, these fatty foods protect good health.

Take eggs. They've been vilified over the years because of their high amounts of saturated fat and cholesterol, but egg yolks—the part of the egg that houses all of the fat and the cholesterol—are rich in antioxidants that protect our eyes and skin against the effects of sunlight and air pollution. These antioxidants are particularly potent at preventing the development of cataracts and macular degeneration, a leading cause of blindness. Eggs are also a phenomenally rich source of choline, a chemical similar to B vitamins, which works with folic acid to reduce levels of homocysteine in the blood. Homocysteine irritates the lining of arteries, making heart disease–causing plaque more likely to form. Choline and other B vitamins (folic acid, B_{12}, and B_6) break down this amino acid into a harmless substance. Beans and cauliflower are also rich in choline, but eggs have 112 milligrams per egg, whereas cauliflower only has 62 per three-quarter cup and beans 48 per half cup. For optimal health, you probably need 425 milligrams of choline a day, which makes starting the day with a three-egg omelet a downright healthful and delicious proposition.

Think avocados are bad for you? Think again. They, along with olives, are loaded with beneficial fats and antioxidants that protect against heart disease and cancer. Both of these foods contain lots of fiber too. Plus, they taste delicious. Eat them guiltlessly. I eat an avocado nearly every day, and I recommend you do the same.

What's not a real food? I could go on for pages, but you can probably guess what I'm about to tell you. Cheez Doodles? Not a real food. Funnel cake? Not a real food. Snickers bar? It's not a real food, but I, for one, wish it was. Fake foods lack the important health-promoting nutrients I just mentioned. Worse, they often contain additives that shorten the life span, reduce energy, and promote cancer. These include:

› **TRANS FATS:** Food manufacturers began using trans fats in the early 1900s to extend the shelf life of foods. Trans fats are what make margarine and Crisco solid at room temperature. They make doughnuts melt-in-your-mouth crispy. They render snack chips into savory and crunchy morsels. They keep most processed foods—like the Twinkie I mentioned—from spoiling *ever*. They make fried chicken finger-licking good, and they are killing us. These fats reduce levels of the good HDL cholesterol and raise levels of the bad LDL cholesterol. This accelerates your risk of having a heart attack or stroke. Trans fats also raise your risk for developing breast cancer, type 2 diabetes, obesity, liver disease, and infertility. These fats are so deadly that you should try to eliminate them from your diet. Shoot for zero consumption of this stuff. Products can claim to be "trans free" even if they have 0.5 grams of the stuff per tablespoon. Always read the list of ingredients. If you see the words *hydrogenated* or *partially hydrogenated*, the product contains trans fats. It's a fake food. Don't buy it.

> **ARTIFICIAL COLORS AND FLAVORS:** How do manufacturers get popcorn to taste like butter, snack chips to taste cheesy, or crackers to taste like chocolate? How do they make foods bright orange or blue or rainbow-striped? They fake it by using a combination of chemicals with names like isoamyl acetate (smells like banana), methyl butyrate (smells like pineapple), and many others. Many foods experts believe that many of these artificial colors and flavors contribute to cancer and overall body aging.

> **SALT:** Excessive salt consumption may raise blood pressure and contribute to stomach cancer. If you ate real food nearly all the time, you wouldn't have to worry about occasionally using your saltshaker to add a little zip to a sliced tomato or cucumber. That's because most people consume most of their salt from processed foods. Read any label from any packaged food: salt is one of the first ingredients. By the way, you should be putting sea salt or kosher salt in your saltshaker. These forms are less processed than typical table salt, and they taste better too.

> **ADDED SUGAR:** Sweeteners from sugarcane and corn (called high-fructose corn syrup) have found their way into nearly every packaged food you'll find at the supermarket, even foods that you probably don't think of as sweet. They not only add unnecessary calories but also contribute to insulin and blood-sugar problems.

BORDERLINE FOODS

So far I've described the easy real foods. Pineapple? Real. Doritos? Fake.

That's child's play. Let's get into the judgment calls. In my opinion, additives, contaminants, and the manufacturing process put the following used-to-be-real foods in the fake-food category.

YOUR EATING SCORECARD

Whether you are following the Real Food Diet or the Skinny Black Dress Diet, I want you to keep track of what you eat every day, your weight, and another factor that's important to you, such as your energy level or mood (use a 1-to-10 scale). This serves two purposes. First, it keeps you honest. If you find yourself fantasizing about crawling under your desk for a nap, you need only look at your scorecard to see why—it was the four glasses of wine you had at the book club last night (not to mention the tiramisu). Second, it helps you pinpoint perfect eating days. On perfect eating days you have no cravings or hunger, you don't feel superstressed about food preparation, and you feel great. Your energy level or mood hits a 10, or you get on the scale the following morning to see a drop in weight.

Here's an example to emulate.

Date: _September 12, 2007_   Weight: _130 pounds_

WHAT I ATE

Breakfast: *Garden Omelet (page 176) with coffee*

Lunch: *Humongous Salad (page 184) with water*

Dinner: *Simplest Ever Poached Salmon (page 195) with steamed broccoli and a side salad, plus a glass of wine*

ENERGY	1	2	3	4	5	6	7	8	9	10
MOOD	1	2	3	4	5	6	7	8	9	10
STRESS	1	2	3	4	5	6	7	8	9	10

CYNTHIA MANN HAIKEN

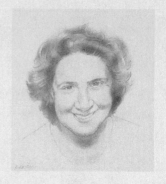

After I gave birth to my second child, my parents gave me a month with Pete as a birthday present. They knew I didn't plan to have more children and that I wanted to get back in shape. They also knew I wasn't a fan of aerobics. I am not a runner and I do not like treadmills or bikes. I don't like dance classes. I don't like any of that stuff. I had never incorporated exercise into a regular routine before. They thought I might like Pete's approach, that I might actually stick with it, and I have.

My first session was easier than I had expected. It wasn't intimidating at all. It was short, and it felt good. Eventually, though, Pete ratcheted up the weights, and the workout became much harder. I learned which machines to dread and which ones would make me want to hurl. To get myself through it, I just kept telling myself that I could do anything *for 90 seconds. Now, even as I walk up to the leg-press machine— my nemesis—I just tell myself that I only have to suffer for 90 seconds. That gets me through it, and in truth, it gives me a tremendous lift to know what I can do. My colleagues, especially my male colleagues, are surprised by the amount of weight that I lift each workout.*

The effect on my body has been noticeable. I used to have these granny arms, and now I have definition in my biceps and triceps. My arms are tighter, and I'm no longer self-conscious about wearing sleeveless shirts, spaghetti straps, or short sleeves. My thighs are tighter too. As much as I hate the leg press, I have to admit that it has really worked! I have more definition in my waist too.

BREAKFAST CEREAL AND OTHER FOODS MADE FROM FLOUR: Most people have to think about this one for a while. Where does breakfast cereal come from? It sure doesn't grow on trees. You can't plant it in a pot and see it take root. Is it a real food? Not quite. Breakfast cereal, crackers, bread, and many other foods come from flour, and flour generally comes from wheat, oats, corn, or soy. Although wheat and other grains are certainly real foods, they lose most of their wholesomeness when they are ground down into flour—even whole grain flour—and used to make packaged foods.

Harvard researchers have been studying the eating habits of thousands of women over many years and have arrived at some startling conclusions about starchy flour-based foods. According to this long-term, well-designed study, diets rich in carbohydrates, particularly foods made from refined flour, promote disease. Consider:

> ›   Women who consumed the highest amounts of starchy carbohydrates were more likely to be diagnosed with infertility than women who consumed the least.

> ›   Women who consumed less carbohydrate and more protein and fat were less likely to develop heart disease, breast cancer, and stroke than women who ate more carbs and less protein and fat.

> ›   Women who ate more starch were more likely to develop gallstones than women who consumed less.

It sure does make one think twice, doesn't it? Here's more. Researchers at the University of Wisconsin–Madison have shown that the tendency for excess carbs—particularly from starch and sugar—to trigger disease and weight gain is wired into our genes. A gene in the liver called SCD-1 (I know, it sounds like R2D2, but you don't need to remember the name of it if you're not inclined to) triggers the body to convert excess carbohydrate calories into fat. If you could switch off this gene—as researchers have done in mice—you could theoretically eat seven loaves of bread a day but wouldn't gain an ounce. Your body wouldn't convert the excess into fat.

Okay, I can almost hear your thoughts again. If you're not thinking it right now, you'll think it eventually. "Pete, isn't breakfast cereal a great way to get my fiber? Isn't it a whole-grain food? Isn't it a great way to get my vitamins and minerals? Ahem, the answers to those questions are short and simple. No, no, and no. High-fiber breakfast cereals are *not* one of the best inventions of modern times. Take a look at the list of ingredients for just about any box of cereal, and you'll find a lot of not-so-real-sounding words and phrases, phrases like:

> Modified corn starch

> Modified wheat starch

> High-fructose corn syrup

> Soy lecithin

> Partially hydrogenated soybean oil

> Artificial flavors

> Artificial colors

> Fractionated palm kernel oil

> Polydextrose

I could go on, but must I? You get the point.

Plus breakfast cereals are made with flour, which is already a refined food, even if it's whole grain. Processors take this flour and compact it under high pressure and high heat to form the hard, thin, crunchy morsels we all know as cereal. This process creates toxins called advanced glycation end products (AGEs), which have been shown to raise levels of harmful free radicals and inflammation in the body, contributing to heart disease, cancer, wrinkles, and overall body aging. Depending on the type and brand, they also add sugar, artificial colors, and flavors to make these crunchy morsels taste, smell, and look appealing, and these artificial colors and flavors may be carcinogenic.

Finally, I've found that many women are sensitive to gluten, a protein in many types of flour. There is nothing more beautiful than a pregnant woman and nothing worse than looking pregnant when you're not. I talk to women all the time who are starving themselves but have protruding bellies. Nine out of ten times, it's the gluten. Found in flour made from wheat, rye, barley, oats, Kamut, spelt, and triticale, this protein can irritate the lining of the small intestine, causing indigestion, gas, fatigue, brain fog, and bloating. Gluten can also have a narcotic effect on some people, triggering intense cravings for sugar and refined foods. Try forgoing flour foods for a week and see what happens. If you feel more energetic and less bloated, you may be sensitive to gluten and should only eat the following grains: corn, brown rice, amaranth, millet, and quinoa.

Bottom Line: I'm not saying that you can never eat bread, cereal, or oatmeal again. I am saying that you should eat real foods in balance. Go for whole foods, especially vegetables (see Rule 2), first. Flour foods should be what you eat if you are still hungry after having vegetables and protein. Whenever you choose foods made from flour, make them as whole as possible (made from whole wheat, oats, or another whole grain).

MILK: Yes, it's a real food. It comes from a cow. Yet the vast majority of people older than age four lack the digestive enzymes (called lactase) needed to break down milk sugar (called lactose), contributing to an endless amount of unnecessary GI distress. If you frequently suffer from gas, bloating, stomachaches, and other GI issues, stop drinking milk and see what happens. If you feel better, you probably cannot digest the lactose.

Even if you are not lactose intolerant, you should probably stop drinking milk. Harvard studies have linked the consumption of lactose with infertility in women. This sugar also raises the risk for ovarian cancer. Finally, the consumption of milk has been shown to worsen acne in teens by affecting hormones.

Bottom Line: Some milk products, such as yogurt and supplemental whey protein, contain very little lactose, so you can consume them without issue. I'm lactose intolerant, and I have no problems with whey protein. I use it five days a week. If you consume dairy, consume only hormone-free dairy products. Most dairy products come from cows that are treated with genetically engineered bovine somatotropin, or rBST, a hormone that increases milk production. This growth hormone can make its way into the milk. When you drink milk with bovine growth hormone, you may increase your risk for developing colon and breast cancers.

CHEESE: Manufacturers make cheese by adding bacteria to milk. The bacteria consume the sugar, reducing the lactose content as they transform the milk into cheese. The problem is that most cheeses have been pasteurized with extremely high heat. This creates the same toxins (called AGEs) found in breakfast cereals. Because cheese comes from milk, some types may also contain hormones that were injected into cattle to boost milk production. These hormones have been linked to estrogen- and progesterone-dependent breast cancers.

Bottom Line: Eat cheese in moderation, no more than three ounces a day. Consume only organic cheeses and if possible purchase them from a local dairy farmer or cheese maker. Because these cheeses go directly from the farm to your refrigerator, they are less likely to be pasteurized under the extremely high heat used for store-bought cheeses. Whenever possible, consume softer cheeses, such as ricotta, which have not been "cooked" as intensely as hard cheeses.

RULE 2:
LOAD UP ON VEGETABLES AND LEGUMES

Think of vegetables and legumes as the foods that counteract your indiscretions. They literally undo the damage caused by bad habits. Pair them with cheese. Pair them with breakfast cereal. Pair them with meat. Pair them with dessert. Consider:

› Beets, broccoli, and spinach are all rich in a nutrient called betaine that helps lower levels of the artery-damaging amino acid homocysteine in the

SIMPLE SOLUTIONS

If you are tired and hungry at dinnertime, you just can't expect yourself to wait twenty or thirty minutes for something to bake in the oven. You'll be into the Doritos before you know it. Ask yourself: What would Wilma eat? I'll tell you. She'd eat the simplest option. The following options provide all of the nutrients you need to steady blood sugar, boost energy, quiet your rumbling stomach, and promote optimal health. Once you get used to eating simply, I'm confident you won't go back to gourmet:

› One to two avocados sliced, pitted, and eaten with a spoon. For a little extra kick, sprinkle a small amount of sea salt or Cajun spice on the avocado. This is a great option on those days when you are too hurried to cook and are considering grabbing fast food. I often have the avocado option when I find myself craving cookies or another dessert or I simply get tired of eating chicken and fish. I eat one or two avocados and I have no desire to eat anything else for the rest of the night, and my cravings for sweets dissolve.

› Sliced veggies with 90-Second Guacamole (page 182).

› 90-Second Ricotta (page 175).

› Three hard-boiled eggs with baby carrots or fruit.

› Strawberry Protein Smoothie (page 181).

› A can of water-packed tuna or wild salmon.

body. In a Harvard study of thousands of nurses, those whose diets were richest in betaine and choline had reduced levels of homocysteine, which protected them from heart disease.

› Most leafy greens are rich in the B vitamin folate, which has been shown to reduce your risk of developing heart disease and to protect against birth defects. Have you heard that alcohol increases your risk of breast cancer? It may be true, and it's also true that folic acid counteracts the effects of alcohol, making that extra glass of wine less likely to cause breast cancer. Beans and lentils also reduce the risk for this cancer.

› Diets high in vegetables and nuts have been shown to reduce the risk of developing gallstones and the need for gallbladder surgery.

› Vegetables and legumes are rich in fiber, which can ease GI distress and reduce your risk of developing colon cancer. They render red meat (see Rule 4) neutral in its effects on the colon. In a Harvard study of more than 30,000 women, people who consumed legumes more than four times a week had a reduced incidence of colon cancer.

› Vegetables and legumes are rich in antioxidant nutrients that fend off carcinogens, reducing your risk for all types of cancer. These antioxidants also prevent eye disease, numb pain, reduce the formation of wrinkles, and protect against memory loss.

Bottom Line: I'm only giving you the following numbers as a ballpark. Aim for more than seven daily servings of vegetables and at least one daily serving of nuts, seeds, beans, or legumes. At every meal and snack, ask yourself, How can I add more vegetables and legumes? Add veggies and beans to omelets. Have a huge salad every day for lunch or dinner. Add them to soup. Try to buy organic produce whenever possible and opt for locally grown produce when it's in season. The more local your produce, the faster it goes from ground to plate and the fewer nutrients it loses in transit.

RULE 3:
DRINK REAL BEVERAGES

Soft drinks? You guessed it. They are not real foods. They're loaded with chemicals such as acetic, fumaric, gluconic, and phosphoric acids, all of which irritate the stomach lining, causing wicked stomachaches. Their carbonation triggers acid reflux, which can eventually irritate the lining of your esophagus and lead to cancer. They contain artificial colors and flavors that may raise the risk for cancer. Finally, they usually contain either high-fructose corn syrup or artificial sweeteners, both of which may raise the risk for diabetes.

You'll get a lot more satisfaction from chewing your calories than from drinking them. Switch to water. If you don't like the taste of water, then try the following options:

> Squeeze lemon or lime into your water.

> Drink iced green, black, or herbal tea.

> Mix a very small amount (no more than one ounce) of 100 percent fruit juice into your water.

Now, I have two surprises that I think you're going to like a lot. First, I'm not against caffeine. Coffee and tea come from plants, which are real foods. Coffee and tea have been shown to reduce your risk of cancer and diabetes. Tea may also strengthen immunity, reduce levels of harmful stress hormones, and protect against memory loss. The antioxidants in tea inhibit bacteria growth in the mouth, working to freshen your breath and protect against gum disease.

Now for the second surprise. I'm not against alcohol, either, *even if you are trying to lose weight*. Alcohol comes from real foods—grapes, in the case of wine, and grain,

Q Should I limit fish because of mercury contamination?

A It's true that fish is contaminated with industrial pollutants such as mercury, dioxin, and PCBs, but a huge, well-done study by Harvard researchers recently showed that the benefits of eating fish far outweigh the risks. Oily fish such as salmon and mackerel contain omega-3 fatty acids, which promote good health, and research shows that eating three ounces of fatty fish a week can reduce the risk of dying from a heart attack by 36 percent and the risk of dying from anything by 17 percent—and that's even if you eat contaminated fish. To reduce levels of contaminants, choose wild salmon most of the time. It's a rich source of omega-3 fatty acids, supplying 1,774 milligrams per six-ounce serving, but tends to be low in contaminants such as mercury, PCBs, and dioxin. Consider the following omega-3 powerhouse fish compared to their levels of contamination:

Fish	Serving	Omega-3s (mg)	Mercury (ppm)	PCBs (ppb)	Dioxin (pg/g)
Wild salmon	6 oz.	1,774	< 0.05	3	.03
Farmed salmon	6 oz.	4,505	< 0.05	21	.5
Anchovy	2 oz.	1,165	< 0.05	n/a	.35
Herring	3 oz.	1,712	< 0.05	n/a	.97
King mackerel	5.4 oz.	1,203	0.05	n/a	.87
Tuna, light	3 oz.	228	0.12	45	.02
Tuna, white	3 oz.	733	0.35	100	.23

in the case of beer. They contain antioxidants that promote good health, and the alcohol itself seems to drive down levels of the bad LDL cholesterol, reduce deadly blood clots, and reduce blood pressure and insulin levels. As a result, moderate drinking has been shown to reduce risks for just about every disease you can name, including heart disease, dementia, Alzheimer's disease, stroke, diabetes, rheumatoid arthritis, gallstones, hearing loss, depression, and certain types of cancer. It even seems to reduce the incidence of the common cold.

But, Pete, you're thinking, won't it make me fat? Well, you know what? That's exactly what I thought, and for years I've been counseling my weight loss clients to lay off the wine. Then my coauthor, a diehard wine lover, put a number of studies in front of me that challenged my belief. Unlike most men, I can admit when I'm wrong, and, in this case, she was right and I was wrong. Reams of research show that moderate drinking does not lead to weight gain, possibly because alcohol tends to speed up the metabolism, causing the body to burn off the excess calories. It also seems to blunt sugar cravings, enabling dieters to automatically eat fewer desserts and other fake foods.

Thing is, some research shows that excessive drinking—more than one drink a day for women—may raise the risk of certain diseases, especially cancer. That's why I want you to hold yourself to one daily drink: a twelve-ounce bottle or can of regular beer, a five-ounce glass of dinner wine, or a shot of liquor or spirits (either straight or in a mixed drink). Also, drink wine with meals rather than before. Drinking wine and other types of alcohol on an empty stomach tends to reduce your inhibitions, causing you to eat many foods that you otherwise would have the willpower to avoid.

Bottom Line: Don't worry about how many glasses of fluid you drink a day. Just drink when you are thirsty and stay away from fake drinks. Consume only water, wine, coffee, and tea.

RULE 4:
LIMIT RED MEAT

Red meat is an exception to my real food rule. Beef, lamb, pork, and other types of red meat have consistently been shown to raise your risk for developing colon, endometrial, and breast cancers, heart disease, high blood pressure, and osteoporosis (weak, brittle bones). It raises the risk for these diseases because it:

STOPS UP YOUR INTESTINES: Red meat takes a long time to digest, and the longer feces sits in your intestines, the longer carcinogens in partially digested food come in contact with intestinal cells.

INTRODUCES TOXINS INTO YOUR BLOODSTREAM: Toxic chemicals called dioxins enter the air from waste incinerators (usually those that burn plastics) and eventually land in water and on grass. Cows and other grazing animals eat grass and consequently they eat this industrial pollutant. Dioxin causes cancer, birth defects, diabetes, learning and developmental delays, endometriosis, and immune system abnormalities. A University of Texas study found that most people have higher blood dioxin levels than the EPA recommends, with more than 90 percent of the exposure coming from food. Because the half-life of dioxin is seven years, dioxin accumulates in animal fat tissue over time, with larger, long-lived animals like cattle containing higher amounts in their meat than smaller, short-lived ones like chickens.

Consider this recent Harvard study of dioxin levels in various foods:

Food	Dioxins in pg/g
Beef	*0.13*
Pork	*0.1*
Mussels	*0.09*
Shrimp	*0.06*

Food	Dioxins in pg/g
Atlantic cod	*0.05*
Eggs	*0.05*
Clams	*0.05*
Wild salmon	*0.03**
Chicken	*0.02*
Tuna, light	*0.02*
Pollock	*0.01*

THROWS OFF HORMONE BALANCE: Estrogen-like hormones are often injected into cattle to fatten them up for slaughter. Unfortunately, what goes in does not necessarily come out. These hormones accumulate in the meat, and studies now show that they tend to trigger early puberty in children and breast cancer in adult women. In a Harvard study that followed more than 90,000 women for many decades, women who ate beef fewer than three times a week were much less likely to develop estrogen- and progesterone-dependent cancers (such as certain types of breast cancer) than women who ate it more often, with risk rising with each additional serving of red meat.

INTRODUCES NITRATES TO YOUR BLOODSTREAM: Nitrates have been linked with lung disease, thyroid dysfunction, and rectal, stomach, throat, and bladder cancers. Nitrates are in nearly all cured foods, including smoked salmon and smoked, cured, or processed meat such as bacon, ham, hot dogs, and deli meat.

CAUSES IRON OVERLOAD: The type of iron (called heme iron) in red meat promotes the formation of nitrates in the GI tract, raising the risk for GI cancers.

Bottom Line: Researchers have linked daily consumption (two or more ounces) of beef, lamb, or pork with an increased risk of disease. Eat red meat no more than twice

---

* Farmed salmon is five times higher in dioxin than beef, due to the dioxin present in the fish feed. Farmed salmon is more than sixteen times higher in dioxin than wild salmon.

a week. If you love red meat, designate one night a week as "red meat night" and follow these tips:

> Make sure any cured meat you purchase is "nitrate free." Many nitrate-free brands are now available.

> Eat only lean cuts of red meat. Pollutants tend to collect in fatty tissue. The leanest cuts are the round, loin, and sirloin for beef, the tenderloin for pork, and the leg, loin roast, and chops for lamb.

> Make sure the red meat you eat is "hormone free." If possible, buy meat locally from a rancher or farmer you trust. It should be raised in pasture and not in a feed lot.

> Cook red meat medium or medium rare to reduce levels of toxins that proliferate when foods are heated. Bonus points: cook meat with water by braising it. This makes it melt-in-your-mouth tender, and the water stops the reaction that causes toxins to proliferate. Avoid grilling, searing, or broiling, as these cooking methods generate carcinogens in the meat.

> Eat meat with plenty of vegetables. The antioxidants and fiber in the veggies will counter the carcinogens and pollutants in the meat. In one study, rats that ate red meat in combination with vegetable fiber did not have colon linings as irritated as rats that ate fiber-free red meat.

REAL FOOD DIET MENU SUGGESTIONS

Use the following menu suggestions to guide your eating.

Breakfast

1. Hot cereal with fruit and 1 ounce chopped nuts.

2. 1/2 melon topped with berries (blueberries, raspberries, blackberries) served with low-fat or fat-free yogurt mixed with 1 tablespoon ground flaxseed or wheat germ.
3. Nicholas's Apple-Banana Shake (page 180).
4. 90-Second Mocha Cappuccino (page 175).
5. Ginger Vegetable Shake (page 176).
6. Strawberry Protein Smoothie (page 181).
7. Leslie's Strawberry-Banana Smoothie (page 180).
8. Garden Omelet (page 176).
9. 90-Second Ricotta (page 175).
10. Carol's Oatmeal Bars (page 200).

Lunch

1. Make your own salad (either prepared at home or at a salad bar):
   › 2 cups lettuce, your choice of vegetables, a palm-size protein (freshly carved chicken breast or grilled fish), 2 tablespoons chickpeas or black beans.
   › For dressing: 2 tablespoons balsamic vinegar, 1 tablespoon olive oil, lemon, salt, and pepper.
2. Bunless turkey or salmon burger topped with salsa and guacamole and served with a side salad.
3. 1 cup ready-made lentil soup (look for low-sodium options) with side vegetable salad.
4. 1 cup ready-made black bean chili topped with chopped onion, plus 1 ounce shredded low-fat cheese with toasted mini whole wheat pita and side of sliced carrots and celery.
5. Carol's Oatmeal Bars (page 200).
6. Tuna Garden Salad (page 196).

7. Pete's Favorite Guacamole (page 192).

8. 90-Second Guacamole (page 182).

9. Alisa's Favorite Stuffed Peppers (page 183).

10. Jennifer's Cali (page 185) or Eastern Burger (page 186) topped with guacamole and served with a side salad.

11. Simplest Ever Avocado Soup (page 193).

Dinner

1. 1 to 2 avocados, eaten with a spoon.

2. Frozen dinner entrée (see the resource list page 203 for recommended options) with side salad.

3. Jennifer's Fish Tacos (page 187) with sliced avocado and a side salad.

4. Jennifer's Cali Burger (page 185) with a side salad.

5. Jennifer's Eastern Burger (page 186) with a side salad.

6. Tuna Garden Salad (page 196).

7. Pete's Favorite Guacamole (page 192).

8. 90-Second Guacamole (page 182)

9. Simplest Ever Poached Chicken (page 194) with baked sweet potato, and steamed broccoli or cauliflower (or 1 cup frozen mixed broccoli/cauliflower).

10. Alisa's Favorite One-Pot Meal (page 182).

11. Marylou's Chicken Soup (page 192) with sliced avocado.

12. Simplest Ever Poached Salmon (page 195) with sautéed spinach and garlic topped with sliced toasted almonds or 1 cup mixed frozen/canned peas and carrots.

13. Simplest Ever Poached Salmon: Almost-As-Simple Variation (page 196) with sautéed spinach and garlic topped with sliced toasted almonds or 1 cup mixed frozen/canned peas and carrots.

14. Leslie's Super Spicy Shrimp Tacos with Black Beans and Brown Rice (page 191).

15. Alisa's Favorite Stuffed Peppers (page 183).

16. Jennifer's Stuffed Peppers (page 188).

17. Simplest Ever Avocado Soup (page 193).

18. Jolynn's As Real As It Gets Pasta (page 190).

PETE'S THREE SIMPLE STEPS FOR EATING OUT

I train New Yorkers. If I told them the only way to eat real was to eat at home, I'd go out of business. Roughly 90 percent of the women I train eat out three meals a day. It can be done. Eating real while eating out is actually very simple. Do the following:

STEP 1: Think about what you will order before you step foot in the restaurant. If possible, get the menu ahead of time. It's a lot easier to make an intelligent ordering decision when you are not smelling and seeing food and when you are not excessively hungry. Tell yourself that you will order lean protein (chicken, turkey, or fish) with vegetables. If it's a special occasion (no more than once a week), allow yourself a red meat dish and give yourself bonus points for ordering a leaner cut such as a sirloin, tenderloin, or filet mignon. Tell yourself that you will stay away from the bread, free crunchy appetizers (tortilla chips, fried wontons, pita with hummus), dessert, and starch (rice, baked potato, etc.). Finally, promise yourself you'll enjoy the conversation and the atmosphere. Take the focus off the food and put it on the experience.

STEP 2: Get to the restaurant and put in your order. If you'd like a glass of alcohol, have it with the meal and not before.

STEP 3: Eat. Okay, so you ate a small dinner roll, a spoonful of dessert, or half a baked potato. I knew you would. I do this all the time. Step 1 and Step 2 are a mind game.

We're all human. If you tell yourself that you will have zero starch and sugar, you'll end up eating only a reasonable amount of the stuff. If you tell yourself, however, that you are going to eat a reasonable amount, you'll probably eat a lot of the stuff. It's mental. In my three-step eating-out approach, the cheating is factored in.

THE SKINNY BLACK DRESS DIET

You're reading this section because you want to lose weight quickly. You want that extra fat off *yesterday*. I get that a lot. I have trained women who have asked me questions like:

> › I'm getting married in three months and I need to fit into my gown. Can you help me?

> › I have a black-tie affair that I have to go to with my husband [or boyfriend] and I can't fit into the dress I bought six months ago. Can you get me into it next week?

Enter the Skinny Black Dress Diet. My Real Food Diet outlined in the previous pages will help you drop pounds, especially if you are a dedicated fake foodie. It won't, however, help you shed fat fast. That's what my Skinny Black Dress Diet does. Thing is, to shed fat fast, you need to work hard. You must work really hard. Think about the intensity of the fitness plan in this book. You'll have to put that same intensity into eating—at least for twenty-four to seventy-eight hours. Yep. That's right. This diet works *that quickly*.

Here's the thing. To put that kind of intensity into eating, you're going to need a very powerful motivational tool. You're going to need a skinny black dress. (It always amazes me that though women are always trying to get into a dress, men are always trying to get them out of them.) It doesn't have to be black and it doesn't even have to be a dress. It just has to be something that you want to get yourself into comfortably in the near future. It can be a pair of skinny jeans. It can be a suit for work. It *can't* be sweats or something with an elastic waistband. I draw the line on clothes that are so forgiving that they allow you to cheat.

So pick your motivational tool. Go to your closet or go shopping and pick out an outfit, one that you want to get into within the next few weeks. Now, get out your calendar. Pick a date to wear your outfit. Schedule it. If it's a skinny black dress, you might make reservations to see an expensive show. If it's skinny jeans, then plan on wearing them to your next book club, night out with your girlfriends, or your kid's Little League game. Just make a date and write it down.

Now here's what I want you to do to get that dress to fit your body. First, you must follow my Four Simple Rules for healthy eating. Okay? Healthy eating is Skinny Black Dress eating. Then tackle the Skinny Black Dress Diet in the following steps.

DRESS DIET STEP 1:
GO LIQUID

In the next few days, you're going to lose four pounds of fat, enough to shrink your body half a clothing size. You'll do it with my twenty-four- to seventy-two-hour Liquid Diet. Before you throw this book against the wall, read on. This really isn't as hard or intense as it sounds. Case in point: when I suggested my coauthor try it after she gained three pounds from a prescription medication, she laughed at me and said, "I'm way too attached to eating to drink my calories for two days. You need to come up with something more realistic." Then she tried it, lost three pounds in just one weekend, and called me the following Monday to report, "You know it really wasn't that bad. I'd do it again."

Whenever I tell people that they can lose up to four pounds in just a couple of days with my Liquid Diet, I invariably hear some smarty-pants science geek say something like, "A pound of fat contains 3,500 calories. There's no way to burn off 14,000 calories in just a few days!"

As I do with any smarty-pants comment, I first pretend I've never heard it before, and, with as much sincerity as I can feign, say, "Oh, I didn't know that. Can you tell me more?" The smarty-pants usually goes on to quote a long list of numbers. She or he might tell me that most people need to eat about 2,000 calories a day to maintain their weight and that even if someone eliminated every single calorie, this would only produce a 6,000 calorie deficit, enough only for a 1.5-pound loss.

Then I do what I always do. I ask her to try it. Three days later she's back at the gym or on the phone, sheepishly telling me, "I don't know how or why it works, but I'm four pounds lighter."

Our bodies are not as precise as calculators. Calories simply don't always add up. You probably know this from experience. There have probably been times in your life when you gained weight even though you knew you were not overeating, and times when you lost weight even though you were not dieting. Both stem from how the body burns fat. When the metabolism is working optimally, it wastes calories, burning fat to produce heat. That's why you can lose three pounds of fat in three days. That's why you can overeat more than a thousand calories at Thanksgiving and not gain an ounce. Your metabolism turns up the heat on fat burning.

That's what my Liquid Diet does. It bathes your body with plenty of fiber, antioxidants, and protein, all designed to kick-start your metabolism. My shake recipes (on pages 176 and 180–81) include plenty of fiber, protein, and fat to keep you full between meals too.

Wait, aren't liquid diets a waste of time? Won't you gain it all back, as Oprah did after she lost weight with Opti-Fast? Oprah regained the weight because she went right back to her bad eating and lifestyle habits after she stopped drinking the shakes. Anyone can gain back weight, and if you do not make permanent lifestyle changes, you will almost certainly regain any weight you lose with the Skinny Black Dress Diet.

Most people, however, *don't* regain what they lose. When researchers from Columbia University analyzed the available studies on liquid meal replacements, they came to only one conclusion: they work. When people lose weight by replacing one or more solid meals with a liquid meal, they tend to lose 7 to 10 percent of their initial weight over three months, compared to only 3 to 7 percent in people who try to cut calories or reduce portion sizes. This improved weight loss lasts as long as a year (the longest study done to date), and people who use the liquid meal replacements are as likely to stick with dieting and maintain their weight loss as people who lose weight through portion control.

Here's how to do it.

For twenty-four to seventy-two hours, consume all of your calories from protein shakes. Your shakes can be as simple as mixing whey powder (check the resources section, page 202, for recommended brands) into a premade vegetable drink and chugging. They can be as complicated as making your own juice with a juicer and then combining the ingredients in a blender. The choice is yours. You'll find a number of my favorite shake recipes on pages 176, 180–81.

Do the Liquid Diet during a string of really busy days. This will keep your mind off food. Who has time to cook when working twelve-hour days? I don't. You'll love that you only need to drink shakes for sustenance.

Tell your loved ones that you will be going on a liquid diet. Tell them that you might need some extra support around the house. Tell them that you'd appreciate it if they didn't eat cookies, candy, and other tempting foods in front of you. Tell them that you'll probably be spending a lot of time relaxing in the bathtub (it's hard to eat cookies when your hands are wet) and that you'll probably go to sleep early. Most important, mention that you may not be your usual chipper self for a few days. Mention that if they dare talk too much or too loudly or at all, you might just bite their heads off. Make a joke out of it. Tell them that you're only biting their heads off because, after two to three days of liquid sustenance, their heads look and smell like chocolate cake.

Q What do you think of artificial sweeteners?

A I highly discourage you from using them. Although the research isn't conclusive, there are enough studies linking enough artificial sweeteners with poor health and undesirable side effects that they should give you pause.

Artificial sweeteners may also cause you to crave what you are trying to avoid: sugar. French research shows that rats actually prefer the intense sweetness of artificial sweeteners to cocaine. The stuff is that addictive. Other researchers suspect that low-calorie sweeteners confuse the brain, allowing it to link sweet flavors with no calories. The problem is that when you eat a high-calorie sweet food, such as ice cream, your brain continues to tell you that you are hungry, even though you've just put away three hundred calories.

Bottom Line: Don't hang out with rats, and don't do what rats do. Do what Wilma did. She didn't use artificial sweeteners. If you must sweeten your foods, I recommend the following:

RAW AGAVE NECTAR: This syrup of the agave cactus contains nutrients called fructans that have been shown in mice studies to induce weight loss and reduce blood cholesterol. The plant also contains sapogenins, a natural antiinflammatory. Agave tastes similar to honey and mixes easily into semisolid or liquid mixtures such as tea, ricotta cheese, plain yogurt, or shakes.

RAW CHOCOLATE: Studies show that chocolate can reduce your risk of heart disease and improve health, but regular processed chocolate is loaded with sugar and cream, both of which add unneeded calories. Raw chocolate, on the other hand, is no more than the actual cacao bean. It's not cooked and it's not mixed with sugar or milk. Some brands mix it with other superfoods such as coconut butter, agave syrup, berries, and nuts. Check out Pete's Instant Craving Stopper (page 201), which combines the good-ness of raw chocolate with agave nectar.

STEVIA: This sweetener is made from a naturally sweet South American herb that is thirty times sweeter than sugar. Remember: I'm into real foods, and stevia is an herb, which means it's real. Studies show that it may act as a natural antioxidant, which protects health and improves blood sugar control. It may even lower blood pressure.

Are you terrified? Don't be. I'm making this sound tougher than it is, and I'm doing that for a reason. I want you to get through the next few days and look back and say to yourself, *Oh, that wasn't as hard as I thought it would be.* The Liquid Diet is similar to the last few seconds of a set during your workout. It's a little uncomfortable, but when you're done, you'll be so proud of yourself, not to mention thrilled with your results.

DRESS DIET STEP 2:
ADD AVOCADO AND GREENS

First things first: get on the scale. How much weight have you dropped? Try on that dress. How does it fit? Okay, you might not be totally in that dress, but you are doing better than four days ago. Do a victory dance. You deserve it.

If you only wanted to drop four pounds, you can move to Step 3. If you still have fat to burn, stay at Step 2 for at least two weeks. When you can't stand eating this way any longer, move to Step 3 as needed, periodically returning to Step 2 and even Step 1 to speed your weight loss. We all need an extra kick of motivation every once in a while that only a big drop on the scale can provide. You'll know when it's time to kick up the effort.

For Step 2, continue to drink that protein shake once a day. You can choose the meal, but I'm going to encourage you to choose breakfast. That's the meal that's most rushed for most people, making a shake a convenient way to kick-start your metabolism for the rest of the day. Now for the other two meals. Choose one of the following:

Option 1. One avocado eaten with a spoon or any of the avocado recipes in chapter 7.

Option 2: The Humongous Salad (page 184)

Yes, it's repetitive. Yes, it's monotonous, and yes, it's crazy effective. I want you to forget everything you've ever heard about the importance of eating a variety of foods. It's hooey. (Note: I wanted to use a different, more manly word from *hooey*, but my coauthor told me that some women would find my language offensive. She said this book is rated PG-13 and she promised to hit me upside the head with said book if I didn't agree with her word choice. I know when to back down.) If you eat real foods most of the time, variety just isn't as important as it is if you are living on Twinkies and Pop-Tarts. Even though Step 2 requires you to eat the same three meals every single day, it provides you with a ton of variety within these meals. You're getting a wealth of vitamins, minerals, antioxidants, and fiber from the salad, avocado, and juice. You're getting a variety of protein from the whey in your shake and the chicken, fish, or egg on your salad.

The avocado, the salad, and the shake are all powerful appetite antidotes. The avocado smothers appetite and cravings with fiber and healthful monounsaturated fat. Both of these ingredients slow digestion. The longer food sits in your stomach and intestines, the longer you feel satisfied after eating and the less your blood sugar fluctuates. Avocado also seems to quiet sugar cravings. I have no true research to prove it but

I know from personal experience and the experiences of hundreds of my clients that an avocado a day keeps the cookie cravings away. The salad further dampens your appetite with even more fiber and lots of water. Vegetables are heavy foods. They weigh down your stomach, quickly inducing the sensation of fullness. Finally, the whey protein in your shake will also slow digestion and steady blood sugar, providing long-lasting fullness.

The shake-avocado-salad diet works for yet another reason. It's boring. That's right, BORING! Eat bananas every day and what happens? You eventually tire of bananas and you naturally eat less. The same goes for nearly any food, including shakes, avocados, and salads. Rather than eating in response to cravings, you eat in response to your body's natural hunger cues.

On the other hand (or fork, if you will), eat many different foods throughout the day and from day to day, and you continually add kindling to your craving furnace. This is why people notoriously overeat at buffet meals and celebratory dinners. They put a little bit of every single option on their plates, and a little bit of everything adds up to a lot of overeating and almost no true satisfaction. Remember the old joke: I'm on the see food diet? Our brains are programmed to make eating feel less pleasurable the longer we eat a specific food. If you eat a plain avocado for dinner, you'll automatically eat less than if you eat a three-course meal or a main course with a number of side dishes. Case in point: in one study, participants were given four courses from combinations of four different foods: sausages, bread and butter, chocolate dessert, and bananas. Some participants were given the same food for each course. Those who had different foods for each course consumed 44 percent more than those who ate the same food for each course.

STEP 3:
INTRODUCE A HOT MEAL

You can't live on avocados, salad, and shakes forever. You're a human being. You dine out. You eat at home with your family. You celebrate the holidays. There will be times in your life when you don't want a shake, don't want an avocado, and don't want to see another salad for as long as you live. I'm with you. I get you, baby.

Here's what I want you to do. Keep your diet as monotonous as possible by following the Dress Diet Menu Suggestions (below) as often as possible. These suggestions will help you to drop up to two pounds a week. As needed, mix in your own recipes and eat-out meals using this one rule: combine lean protein and lots of vegetables. In the Real Food Diet, you'll see that I'm not big on cutting fat. You're trying to lose weight, however, and cutting fat allows you to fill up on a higher volume of food with much fewer calories. For weight loss, opt for egg whites, skinless poultry, fish, shellfish, and part-skim or low-fat yogurt and cheese. You can eat as much lettuce, spinach, cabbage, carrots, peppers, cucumbers, and other vegetables as you like.

In the following pages you will find my recommended menu options for breakfast, lunch, and dinner. Choose from these recommended foods *most of the time*. They are all low in craving-inducing refined carbs and high in appetite-suppressing protein and fiber.

Dress Diet Menu Suggestions

Breakfast Options

1. Protein shakes (starting on page 175 for various recipes).
2. Garden Omelet (page 176) made with egg whites.

Lunch Options

1. 1 avocado eaten with a spoon.
2. The Humongous Salad (page 184).
3. Bunless turkey or salmon burger topped with salsa and guacamole and served with a side salad.

Dinner Options

1. Avocado night: 1 avocado eaten with a spoon, guacamole (pages 182 and 192 for recipes), Alisa's Favorite Stuffed Peppers (page 183), or Simplest Ever Avocado Soup (page 193).
2. Simplest Ever Poached Chicken (page 194) with steamed broccoli or cauliflower (or 1 cup frozen mixed broccoli/cauliflower).
3. Simplest Ever Poached Salmon (page 195) or its Almost-as-Simple Variation (page 196) with sautéed spinach and garlic topped with sliced toasted almonds or 1 cup mixed frozen/canned peas and carrots.
4. Frozen dinner entrée (see the resource lists on page 202 for recommended options) with side salad.

STEP 4:
MAINTAIN WITH THE REAL FOOD DIET

So the dress fits! Congratulations. Let's keep it on you. To ensure you can fit into it for the rest of the year—for the rest of your life—start following my Real Food Diet for good health with one modification. Keep your protein lean. Continue to weigh yourself daily. This will keep you accountable to those times when you cheat—say, having nachos and three beers in one evening. If you gain a few pounds, just go to Step 1 of the Dress Diet and get them right back off. Then return to the Real Food Diet with renewed commitment.

SIMPLY EAT, SIMPLY SAVOR

In an ideal world, you'd be able to fuel your body with all of the elements of good nutrition with your knife and fork. This isn't a perfect world. Modern farming practices have rendered fruits and vegetables not as nutritious as they were in years past. Chronic stress, lack of sleep, and an on-the-go lifestyle tax the body in ways that solid food can't always fix. To be optimally healthy, you need supplements. Turn the page to learn how to save money on them.

CHAPTER 4

Save Money on Supplements

My only personal interest in the supplements I recommend involves you and your health. I want you to sleep more deeply, feel more relaxed, have more energy, and live a longer, happier, healthier life, and to reap those benefits, you need a few supplements.

I'm talking about as few as three and as many as five, depending on your lifestyle, health, and age. Research consistently shows that most of us—including the healthiest of eaters—are deficient in something. A Harvard review of the available studies determined, "Most people do not consume an optimal amount of all vitamins by diet alone." If you don't take supplements, you probably won't get a deficiency disease such as scurvy or beriberi, but less-than-optimal amounts of specific vitamins and minerals can leave you vulnerable to developing heart disease, osteoporosis (thinning of the bones), and some cancers.

In the following pages, you'll find my "must take" list of supplements.

Check with your doctor before taking any supplements, especially if you are taking prescription medicines. I recommend the following supplements daily:

IN THE MORNING:

1. Multivitamin mineral supplements that contains roughly 100 percent of the Daily Value (DV) for most vitamins and minerals
2. Optional: Vitamin C, 400 mg to 1000 mg
3. Optional: B Complex
4. Fish Oil: 400 mg to 2 grams

AT NIGHT BEFORE BED:

5. 5-HTP: 50 mg

MULTIVITAMIN/MINERAL

LOOK FOR: *A product bearing the U.S. Pharmacopeia Dietary Supplement Verification Program (USP-DSVP) mark that contains roughly 100 percent of the daily value (DV) for most vitamins and minerals. It should not exceed the upper limit in vitamins and minerals that could become toxic, as listed on page 126.*

Your multivitamin/mineral supplement fills most of the nutritional gaps in your diet. Think of it as an insurance policy. You may never really need it, but it's there for you on those occasional days when you don't eat as well as you should. Two factors make it more likely that you will need to repeatedly cash in on this insurance policy. First, the practice of harvesting produce before it ripens and trucking it thousands of miles over multiple days to a grocery store near you adds up to one problem: nutrient loss.

The longer it takes for a fruit or vegetable to go from stalk to plate, the more nutrients it loses. You can minimize some of these losses by purchasing locally grown produce that is picked at the peak of the ripening cycle or by choosing frozen produce during the winter months if local produce is not available. Second, strength training, stress, and lack of sleep all raise your needs for vitamins and minerals.

According to researchers, the most important vitamins and minerals include:

> B vitamins, especially B_6 and B_{12}: low levels raise your risk of heart disease and breast cancer, and the intestines are less able to absorb these vitamins as you age.

> Vitamin D: increasingly D is being touted as the new wonder vitamin, and for good reason. A lack of D in the diet has been linked to colon and breast cancer, tuberculosis, schizophrenia, multiple sclerosis, hip fractures, and chronic pain. Most tissues and cells in the body use the vitamin, including your bones. In fact, D may be even more important than calcium in keeping your bones strong. As you get older, your skin does not make vitamin D as effectively, and sunscreens (which are a must to prevent skin cancer and wrinkles) block vitamin D production altogether. The average person consumes only about 230 International Units (IU) through food, but research suggests we need about 1,500 IU.

> Antioxidant vitamins A, C, and E: by neutralizing age-promoting free radicals, these important age stoppers reduce your risk of many different diseases, including heart disease, diabetes, and cancer. Our bodies do not absorb these antioxidants efficiently as we get older. You probably need to consume nine or more servings of produce to get enough antioxidants in your system. That's the equivalent of four and a half cups of vegetables a day. If you're not consuming that much, a multivitamin that contains this trio of antioxidants is a must.

Look for a multi that provides at least 100 percent of the DV for vitamins A, C, D, E, K, and all B vitamins. Solgar VM75 is a great choice. I have no affiliation with this company, by the way. I recommend its multi because I take it myself and it has a proven track record. It contains at least 100 percent of the important vitamins and minerals. If you'd like to purchase a different brand or check your current brand against the DVs, use the chart below for comparison. Many supplements, including the Solgar brand provide much more than the DV for some nutrients. This is a good thing. The DVs list the nutrient amounts you need to prevent malnutrition. You probably need more than the DV in specific nutrients—especially vitamin C, vitamin D, and B vitamins—to ensure optimal health.

A few vitamins can be toxic in high amounts. For those vitamins, I've included the upper limit. You should make sure your supplement contains less than this maximum amount.

VITAMIN	DAILY VALUE	UPPER LIMIT
A	5,000 IU	10,000 IU
B_1 (thiamin)	1.5 mg	
B_2 (riboflavin)	1.7 mg	
B_3 (niacin)	20 mg	35 mg
B_5 (pantothenic acid)	10 mg	
B_6 (pyridoxine)	2 mg	100 mg
B_7 (biotin)	300 mcg	
B_9 (folic acid)	400 mcg	
B_{12} (cobalamin)	6 mcg	
C	60 mg	2,000 mg
D	400 IU	2,000 IU
E	30 IU	1,000 mg
K	80 mcg	

VITAMIN C

LOOK FOR: *A separate supplement with about 400 milligrams per day if you are in good health. If you are under a lot of stress (three full-time jobs and a cranky baby), take 1,000 milligrams. If you are fighting a cold, take 2,000 milligrams (1,000 milligrams twice a day) until your symptoms resolve.*

Most multivitamins contain more than the DV for vitamin C (also known as ascorbic acid), and for most people that's enough, especially if you are consuming plenty of vitamin C–rich fruits and vegetables. If you have joint issues, are under a lot of stress, or have been diagnosed with heart disease, diabetes, or another age-related disease, then I recommend you supplement your multi with a vitamin C supplement. In a study of 293 adults, higher vitamin C intake was associated with reduced incidence of bone marrow lesions, a common source of pain in people with osteoarthritis. Supplemental vitamin C may also slow aging as a result of its antioxidant effect. Vitamin C protects molecules all over the body—including proteins, fats, and DNA—from free radical damage. It has been shown to prevent just about every disease. Consider the following:

> › Vitamin C supplements—ranging in dose from 250 milligrams to 1 gram a day—have been shown to increase immunity in marathoners, skiers, and soldiers, halving the incidence of the common cold. Other studies show that vitamin C shortens the duration of a cold by 8 percent, or about two days.

> › Low intakes of vitamin C raise risk for heart disease, and high intakes lower risk. The First National Health and Nutrition Examination Study (NHANES I) Epidemiologic Follow-up Study completed by the University of California at Los Angeles determined that the risk of dying from a heart

attack was 42 percent lower in men and 25 percent lower in women who consumed about 300 milligrams of C a day through food and supplements. The ongoing Nurses Health Study of more than 85,000 women yielded similar results, revealing a 28 percent drop in heart disease risk with vitamin C intakes above 359 milligrams a day.

› This vitamin can protect blood vessels in your brain too. A twenty-year study of two thousand Japanese residents found that risk of stroke was 29 percent lower in people with the highest blood levels of vitamin C.

› People who consume more vitamin C tend to have reduced rates of mouth, throat, vocal cord, esophageal, lung, stomach, colon, and rectal cancers, with risk reductions as high as 64 percent.

› Vitamin C concentrates in the lens of the eye, where it shields cells and molecules from UV damage. People with low levels of vitamin C in this part of the eye or whose diets are low in C tend to have a higher incidence of cataracts.

B VITAMINS

LOOK FOR: *I like the brand Solgar B-Complex "50." Each capsule has 50 milligrams of thiamin, 50 milligrams of riboflavin, 50 milligrams of niacin, 50 milligrams of vitamin B_6, 400 micrograms of folic acid, 50 micrograms of vitamin B_{12}, 50 micrograms of biotin. Take one capsule most of the time, but if you are so stressed that you fantasize about stabbing your spouse with a butcher's knife, increase your dosage to two capsules.*

I recently counseled a woman whose child was struggling in school. Her husband was no help, and work was a bit overwhelming. As a result, she was grinding her teeth at night and repeatedly visiting her internist with vague symptoms such as muscle aches and spasms. Nothing he prescribed seemed to help. When she told me about it, I asked her whether she was taking a B complex supplement. She wasn't. She started, and within a few weeks all of her symptoms resolved. She told me she felt younger and more resilient. "Hey, I'm just trying to give you enough ammo to deal with your normal life," I replied.

If you work too much, play too much, family too much, and sleep too little, or you are going through a stressful transition (buying a home, adjusting to a new job, going through a divorce), I recommend you add a B complex supplement. What is B complex? It's a group of the following eight vitamins:

Thiamine (B_1)
Riboflavin (B_2)
Niacin (B_3)
Pantothenic acid (B_5)
Pyridoxine (B_6)
Cyanocobalamin (B_{12})
Folic acid
Biotin

These eight vitamins work together to support metabolic and muscular function, promote healthy skin, improve immunity and nerve function, and promote cell growth and division. B vitamins may be particularly important in battling the effects of stress. The stress hormone cortisol depletes B vitamins. (By the way, the stress response also depletes vitamin C.) Consider:

> ›   Your body needs optimal amounts of vitamin B_6 to make the soothing brain chemical serotonin from the amino acid tryptophan. This is why you can feel depressed or anxious if vitamin B_6 levels drop too low.

> Immunity tends to drop when we're under stress, which is why most people tend to get a bout of the common cold when they can least afford to deal with it. (Life is cruel that way, isn't it?) Vitamin B$_6$ helps to prevent this stress-induced drop in immunity by supporting immune system cells called lymphocytes and a protein called interleukin-2. Vitamin B$_2$ also enhances your body's resistance to bacterial infections.

> A March of Dimes study of 1,355 pregnant women determined that life stress increased the incidence of birth defects such as spina bifida (exposed spinal cord) and anencephaly (exposed brain and absence of a forebrain), especially in women who did not take folic acid supplements.

> In addition to protecting your body from the effects of stress, B vitamins prevent both heart disease and cancer, particularly breast and colon cancers. B$_6$, folic acid, and B$_{12}$ are important in controlling levels of homocysteine, a harmful blood chemical that raises the risk for heart disease and stroke. This trio of B vitamins helps to convert homocysteine back into cysteine or methionine, both of which are harmless.

FISH OIL

LOOK FOR: *If you are healthy, take a supplement that contains 400 to 600 milligrams a day of combined EPA (eicosapentaenoic acid) and DHA (docosahexaenoic acid), the two main fatty acids in fish, with no more than twice as much EPA as DHA. If you have heart disease or a family history of developing it, or you are recovering from an injury, take 1 to 2 grams a day. Consult your physician if you are taking a medication that increases bleeding, blood pressure medicine, diabetes medicine, or cholesterol-lowering medicine. If your fish oil smells fishy, it's not a good-quality supplement. Look for labeling on* *the packaging or call the company to determine whether your supplement has gone through molecular distillation and ultrafiltration, both of which remove impurities such as mercury as well as fishy scent. Store your fish oil in the refrigerator.*

As I mentioned in chapter 3, fish—even if it is contaminated with pollutants—slows aging and promotes good health. Fish oil supplements are one better because they have been purified. They provide you with all of the beneficial health-promoting omega-3 fatty acids without the dioxin, mercury, and PCBs. Consumer Lab, an independent supplement testing company, found all of the supplements it tested were free of contaminants such as mercury.

Our bodies evolved on diets rich in omega-3 fatty acids, the type of fat found abundantly in cold water fish such as salmon. Early humans ate roughly the same amount of this type of fat as they did omega-6 fatty acids (the type of fat found in grains, vegetable oils, and nuts). Today, however, we eat twenty times as much omega-6 as we do omega-3. Although omega-6 fats are not necessarily bad for us, this imbalance between the two types of fats tends to increase inflammation in the body, triggering the immune system to attack healthy tissue such as your blood vessels, brain cells, joints, and muscle mass.

Taking a fish oil supplement helps

GET YOUR MONEY'S WORTH

Studies completed by a number of independent testing labs have revealed a depressing trend: many supplements don't contain the vitamins, minerals, and other nutrients that they advertise. To get your money's worth, make sure any supplement you purchase contains a seal from the United States Pharmacopeia (USP). This independent public health authority sets public standards for all over-the-counter medicines and screens participating supplement companies for ingredient integrity, purity, and potency.

to shift this balance in the right direction. As a result, high consumption of fish or fish oil supplements has been shown to reduce heart disease, stroke, and age-related macular degeneration (a leading cause of blindness). Fish oil has also been shown to boost mood, and it may help control body weight. Your supplement will help you to:

> **EAT LESS:** A Mayo Clinic study determined that African tribes who consumed a fish-rich diet had lower levels of the hormone leptin, indicating that their brains were probably less resistant to its effects. Although leptin is considered a satiety hormone—one that turns off appetite—higher levels are not necessarily a good thing. Fat cells secrete leptin. The more fat cells you have and the more fat those cells store, the more leptin they secrete. As leptin levels go up, brain cells stop responding to it by turning off appetite. Fish oil may sensitize brain cells, making them more responsive to leptin and allowing the hormone to flip off your appetite switch more easily.

> **FEEL HAPPIER:** A Taiwanese review of ten different studies of people with mood disorders determined that supplementing with omega-3 fatty acids significantly lifted mood.

> **LIVE LONGER:** Fish oil may protect against heart disease by stabilizing plaque (making it less likely to rupture and form a clot), normalizing heart rhythm, and reducing triglycerides and blood pressure. An Emory University review of research determined that omega-3 fatty acid supplements reduced risk of death from heart attack by 36 percent and overall risk of dying from *any* disease by 17 percent.

> **REDUCE PAIN:** A York University (Canada) review of seventeen studies determined that fish oil supplements significantly reduced joint pain intensity,

minutes of morning stiffness, the number of painful joints, and the need to consume painkillers.

> **IMPROVE EXERCISE RECOVERY:** Research completed by the Center for Genetics in Washington, D.C., determined that fish oil consumption helped to reduce postexercise inflammation, encouraging muscles to recover more quickly.

Got kids? Consider having them take supplements as well. Studies show that children with learning disabilities, problems focusing, and hyperactivity issues all benefit from fish oil. I give it to my kid. My ten-year-old son, Nicholas, has some difficulties focusing in school, and, as a parent, I want to do anything and everything for him. When I read the studies about how fish oil was helping children with learning disabilities, I ran out and got a bottle that day. I figured I had nothing to lose and everything to gain. If it didn't help his focusing issue, it would at the very least make him healthier and get him into a great habit. Buy a product designed for children and follow package directions for dosage.

Ask Pete

Q I understand that fish oil is good for me, but I'm a vegetarian. Is there a plant-based way to get my omega-3s?

A You can, but it's a lot harder to consume therapeutic amounts of omega-3s from plants than from fish. Fish oil comes in a form of omega-3 that the body can easily use. The body must convert the type of fat in plant foods such as flaxseeds and walnuts to EPA. Only about 5 percent of the fat in plant foods gets converted into the usable form of omega-3s. Go ahead and take a flaxseed oil supplement, and consume walnuts, ground flax, and beans—all omega-3-rich plant foods—often. To help your body convert plant fat into a form it can use, take your flax supplement at the same time you take your multivitamin, vitamin C, and B vitamins. Cut back as much as possible on trans fats, cooking oils, and alcohol, as they all tend to block the omega-3 conversion.

5-HTP

LOOK FOR: *A supplement that contains 50 milligrams. Increase to 100 milligrams only if needed. This supplement interacts with some prescription medications. Consult your physician before taking 5-HTP if you are taking any prescription medicine.*

Most of the women I train can only find time for themselves by skimping on the one thing they need most—sleep. Our high-paced, high-stress lifestyles are causing more sleep disorders than ever before. In addition, melatonin—the sleep hormone—declines with age, reducing sleep efficiency. Menopause also tends to worsen sleep, and research shows that menopausal women are more likely to have insomnia.

Without enough sleep, our muscles do not recover from exercise and our hormonal levels become unbalanced, leading to an overactive appetite. Studies consistently show that people who sleep less tend to have higher levels of the hunger hormone ghrelin and lower levels of the satiety hormone leptin.

That is where 5-HTP (5-hydroxytryptophan) comes in. In the body, this amino acid is converted into serotonin, a brain chemical that induces calmness. The brain converts this chemical into the sleep-inducing melatonin. (By the way, this amino acid is also found in turkey, which it is one reason why many people feel sleepy after Thanksgiving dinner.)

5-HTP is used to treat many conditions related to serotonin deficiency, including depression, binge eating, chronic headaches, and insomnia. A study of fifty patients with fibromyalgia in Italy found that patients who took 5-HTP had improved sleep, were less anxious, and had reduced pain and stiffness. 5-HTP may also lift mood, reduce anxiety, dampen appetite, and numb pain.

ONLY WHAT YOU NEED

Now you've come to the end of the chapter. If you're a woman older than thirty-five, you're probably thinking, But Pete, what about calcium? I'm not going to tell you not to take calcium, but I will tell you that vitamin D is probably more important for bone health. Experts at Harvard and other highly respected institutions have been questioning whether the Institute of Medicine's recommendation of 1,000 to 1,500 daily milligrams of calcium is just too high. Some research suggests that calcium supplements do no good, and at least one study found that the bones of women who took calcium supplements got weaker over three years than the bones of women who did not take a supplement. Why the conflicting results? Your bones need minerals like calcium to stay strong. There's no doubt about that, but if you don't stimulate your bones with strength training or another type of weight-bearing exercise, your bones have no incentive to strengthen themselves. You could take a million calcium pills a day, but without stimulation, your bones will ignore a lot of this calcium. Also, if you smoke, drink too much alcohol (more than one drink a day), take certain types of prescription medications, and do too much cardio (you're a marathoner, for example), your body will excrete a lot of the calcium you consume.

It seems prudent to load up on calcium-rich real foods (dark green leafy vegetables such as kale and broccoli are powerhouses), do weight-bearing exercise such as strength training to stimulate bone mineral absorption, and avoid lifestyle activities known to weaken bones (such as smoking, excessive drinking, and excessive exercise).

Again, I'm not telling you to stop taking your calcium supplement. I'm just trying to give you all of the facts and I'm trying to save you money. If you are already taking calcium, keep it up. If you are not, it's a good idea to have a nutritionist analyze your nutrition scorecard. A registered dietitian can look at your food log to see just how much calcium you're consuming through your diet. Chances are, if you follow my Real Food Diet as directed, you're getting all of the calcium you need.

My supplement plan, my eating plan, and my exercise plan all share one thing in common: they ask no more of you than what you really and truly need to look and feel your best. Three to five supplements at a cost of less than $10 a month? You can do this. Get on the Internet. Go to the vitamin store. Stock up, and then turn to the next chapter to find the final ingredient in the 90-Second Fitness Solution.

CHAPTER 5

Stress-Proof Your Life

It seems as if space always gets filled up. If you move to a bigger house, you buy new furniture and more knickknacks and eventually need an even bigger house. If you get a raise, your expenses grow and your savings account doesn't. (Usually it dwindles as your income goes up!) If you have kids, you don't work less to make time for your family. No, you still work sixty hours a week and you care for your family too. If you don't have a family, then you fill the time by working an extra forty hours and rewarding yourself by partying (and exhausting yourself further) on the weekends.

Either way, we all seem to fill in the space, and the lack of space is killing us. I see it all the time—the dark circles under the eyes, the blank stares, the lack of results from exercise, the excessive cravings for sugar, the anxiety, the insomnia, the afternoon slump, the moodiness, the reduced immunity, and the forgetfulness. (*I walked into this room for a reason, didn't I?*) The time and determination you put into these lifestyle changes must come from somewhere, and that means some of the clutter that is filling up your brain and your life must go.

Create more space at home, at work, and in your body by:

› Doing just one task at a time.

› Never putting more than seven tasks on your daily to-do list and always allowing one task to wait until tomorrow.

› Sleeping no more and no less than your body needs, using your daytime drowsiness as a gauge.

› Spending five minutes cleaning out a small area of your home or office on the days you work out.

› Using Pete's Life Balance Sheet (page 150) to keep life simple.

My Stress-Proofing Life Plan is about making space—space in your closet, space in your kitchen cabinets, space in your desk drawers, and space in your psyche. As you create more space—by doing, buying, and thinking *less*—you'll get more energy, more bliss, more calm, and more control.

MAKE HEAD SPACE

Trying to do two tasks at once usually means you'll do one or both of them poorly. Yes, that's right: multitasking—the time-saver of the new millennium—wastes more time than it saves. Research done at the University of Michigan has determined that office workers get more done more quickly if they stick with one task at a time. Those who split their time between their computer, their BlackBerry, and their landline get the least done in a day. Consider the following:

> People who talk on their cell phone—even if it's hands-free—while driving are more likely to get into accidents and less likely to pay complete attention to their phone conversation.

> People who eat in front of the computer or the TV put away more calories than people who eat at a dining room table.

It takes our brains a few seconds to switch from one task to another. It's similar to using two computers at once. As you use one computer, the screen saver flips on the other. Then you go to the other and have to wait a few seconds to interrupt the screen saver and warm up the computer. Our brains work the same way. In the end, you'll get more done if you do only one thing at a time.

Bottom Line: Go ahead and check e-mail while you are in a bus or taxi. In that case, you are saving time. Don't do it while driving, talking on the phone, or cooking. For the sake of your relationship, keep your iPhone or BlackBerry out of the bedroom.

MAKE CALM SPACE

We all have some stress. If you had none, you'd probably have a hard time getting out of bed in the morning. Stress becomes overwhelming, however, when your stress response—the heightened muscle tension, rapid heart rate, and sweaty palms—continually overrides your relaxation response so that you rarely, if ever, experience a state of calm.

A chronically activated stress response interferes with sleep. Stressed people tend to wake more than calm people and do not sleep as deeply, according to University of Pittsburgh research.

Stress also depletes the body, reducing your ability to fight infections. Too much stress also contributes to all of the diseases that sleep deprivation does, raising your risk for heart disease, cancer, and diabetes. Stress can even cause your skin to break out. In one study completed at Wake Forest University School of Medicine, teens under high stress were 23 percent more likely to suffer more pronounced and more frequent acne breakouts than teens with less stress.

Do I need to cite more research to prove to you that getting stressed out over your to-do list is a colossal waste of your time? Here are some simple ways to switch off your inner taskmaster:

PICK UP THE PACE WHEN YOU DO YOUR CARDIO: Cardio is optional on the 90-Second Fitness Solution, but if you love to power walk, run, cycle, or something else, then make more space by doing it intensely. Research at the University of Missouri-Columbia shows that high-intensity exercise—the kind that makes you breathe hard and sweat—helps drive down stress and anxiety better than low-intensity exercise such as casual walking, especially for women. So if you are having a tough week, do the elliptical workout described on page 84, or pick up the pace during your usual cardio, alternating hard one-minute bursts with an easier pace for one minute.

LAUGH: Laughter is one of the fastest ways to reduce stress and anxiety. When you are feeling tense, call a friend who makes you laugh, read the comics, or find a funny video to watch on YouTube. You might even sign up for a joke-of-the-day daily e-mail.

GIVE YOURSELF QUIET TIME EVERY DAY: Life is filled with noise. It seems everywhere you go, your ears are bombarded with Muzak, traffic, construction, and mindless chatter about the weather. Once a day, give yourself some quiet. Turn off the TV and radio. Unplug the phone. Turn off the pager and cell phone. Go to your own personal hideaway. It might be your bedroom or a sunny room in your house. It might be a quiet spot at work where no one bothers you. It might be somewhere out in nature.

If you're in a public place, do yourself a favor by wearing headphones attached to a CD player or iPod. Don't turn on the music though. The headphones will drown out the noise of the other conversations around you and they'll make people think twice before talking to you. (Just don't wear them while having sex!) If you are at work, you can do the same with a headset attached to a phone.

Hang out in your quiet zone for five to ten minutes. You might sip some tea, read a novel or magazine, or simply sit and stare into space. What you do during your quiet time is up to you, as long as you take the time to unplug from the world, and particularly the world's electronic and battery-powered devices.

GET BUSY—IN THE BEDROOM: It's physically impossible to be stressed out while experiencing sexual pleasure. The part of the brain that worries—called the amygdala—must switch off for the rest of the brain to fire up those sexual feelings. Plus, there's nothing quite like a deep lovemaking session—even if it's a quickie—to calm you down, put life in perspective, and ensure you have a nice smile on your face.

INDULGE YOURSELF: Sign up for a massage, take a yoga or tai chi class, or get a pedicure. Allow yourself whatever extravagance in time or cost that you normally would think of as a splurge. Massages, whether from a professional or a friend, are particularly effective for releasing muscle tension. You are worth it. Make yourself and your peace of mind your number-one priority.

Bottom Line: You are the boss of your time and energy. Never put more than seven tasks on your daily to-do list, and always allow one task to wait until tomorrow. If you have the choice between completing one more task or giving yourself a little extra unstructured space, take the space. I believe in the opposite of J. A. Spender, the guy who said, "Never put off until tomorrow what you can do today." Pete says, "Never do today what you can put off until tomorrow. Procrastination rules!"

MAKE A RESTING SPACE

Early humans evolved without indoor lighting, flashlights, and window treatments. As a result, they hunted and gathered during daylight and they relaxed and slept at night. Our bodies evolved with this pace, and these millions of years of evolution have given us bodies that function with varying day-and-night cycles. Our brain cells contain pacemakers or little clocks that direct body temperature, hormone release, brain chemical production, stress response, metabolism, and even fat burning to fluctuate from night to day.

Thanks to these pacemakers, our sleep follows a predictable pattern. You lie down, you close your eyes, and you drift off into slow-wave sleep. Growth hormone rises, causing cells throughout your body to slow down and rest. Body cells use less blood sugar to burn for energy, slowing metabolism. The pancreas makes less of the hormone insulin. Everything slows down. As dawn breaks, levels of the stress hormone cortisol rise, triggering cells throughout your body to wake up and resume normal metabolism. End result: you wake refreshed.

At least, that's what *should* happen. That's what *would* happen if we didn't disrupt our natural internal cycles by keeping ourselves awake long past sunset—through the use of indoor lighting, television, and computers, and by waking ourselves before daybreak with the use of the alarm clock. More people were sleeping fewer than six hours in 2004 than in 1985. In 1960 most people slept between eight and nine hours at night, but by 1995 time spent sleeping dropped to seven hours. More than 30 percent of women aged thirty to sixty-four now sleep fewer than six hours. But at least we now have cable.

Most people compensate for one night of sleep deprivation by sleeping longer and more deeply the next night. After repeated nights of deprivation, however, the body seems to adjust to the sleep loss, with hormones shifting to drive up appetite *and* interfere with sleep. This is why sometimes you can't fall asleep or stay asleep even though you feel dead tired. You're actually too tired to sleep.

This type of chronic sleep deprivation has been linked with everything that could possibly ail you, including obesity, diabetes, metabolic syndrome, and heart disease. Even if you sleep eight hours—but do so during the day rather than at night—you mess around with your body's internal clock and suffer unfortunate consequences as a result. Shift workers, for example, tend to be heavier than people who sleep at night, and they have higher rates of gastrointestinal problems, heart disease, and diabetes. In hamsters a nocturnal lifestyle shortens life span.

Just a few days of sleep deprivation is enough to reduce insulin sensitivity and drive up blood sugar. And I'm not just talking about a little dip in sensitivity or bump in blood sugar. I'm talking about an increase in blood sugar that is similar to the early stages of diabetes. Chronic sleep loss has even been linked to poor eyesight.

In addition to shortening your life span, sleep loss also makes you fat. Mild sleep deprivation—say, sleeping for only six hours at night instead of eight—is enough to increase levels of the hunger hormone ghrelin by 15 percent. Researchers estimate that this increase in hunger triggers the consumption of an extra 350 to 500 calories a day, enough to cause you to gain up to one pound a week.

Lack of sleep also chronically raises levels of the stress hormone cortisol, making you feel on edge during the day and more susceptible to stress-induced eating. It also makes you feel too fatigued to do your workout. Finally, it makes you stupid. Just try to have a conversation with me if I've been up all night with my eight-month-old. I'm an idiot! Studies show that mild amounts of sleep deprivation cause deficits in all sorts of cognitive functions, including higher-order executive functions, emotional intelligence, constructive thinking, intrapersonal functioning, assertiveness, sense of independence, empathy, stress management skills, impulse control, and behavioral coping. In laywomen's terms? When you are sleep deprived, you are less likely to ask for what you need, communicate effectively, or help others. You are also more likely to tell off your boss, snap at loved ones, tailgate, curse (hell yeah!), and eat ice cream straight from the container. Did you just read that last sentence and say: Oh my god! That's me!? Me too.

Sleep should create space, but when you sleep too little or too inefficiently it steals space by souring your mood, inducing fatigue, and making you sick. If, according to your Simple Sleep Scorecard (page 143), you are getting enough sleep, then I give you advanced placement credits. If your scorecard reveals sleep debt, use one or more of my simple sleep prescriptions until you earn yourself a passing grade on the scorecard:

TAKE SHORT NAPS DURING THE DAY: A fifteen- to twenty-minute midafternoon nap can help you shorten your sleep deficit, according to Japanese research. Just don't sleep longer than twenty minutes. That will allow you to get into the deeper stages of sleep, which are more difficult to wake from and may interfere with sleep at night.

DIM THE LIGHTS: Too much artificial light at night tricks your brain into thinking that it's still daytime, throwing off melatonin production. I don't expect you to live like a cavewoman—rummaging around in darkness—but it's not a bad idea to turn down lighting as much as possible at sunset. If possible, put overhead lighting on dimmer switches and completely turn off any unnecessary lighting. Consider using candles. They are calming and get you into the perfect state of mind for sleep. In the hour before bed, turn off your TV and computer. Both emit light and radiation, which can prevent the rises in melatonin needed for sleepiness at bedtime.

WATCH SITCOMS: If you watch TV in the evening, opt for sitcoms rather than dramas. Research shows that laughter increases melatonin production. In a study done on forty children with dermatitis (an itchy skin rash), watching a funny movie before bed reduced the number of times the children woke at night.

TAKE A WALK AFTER DINNER: Exercise of any kind has been shown to improve sleep, but Japanese research shows that small amounts of daily exercise are best, especially in the early evening.

HAVE CAFFEINE IN THE MORNING, NOT IN THE AFTERNOON: Caffeine produces alertness by blocking sleep-inducing chemicals and increasing stress hormones. Caffeine's half-life is six hours, which means some caffeine is in your system twelve or more hours after you've had that cup of coffee, and it's still keeping levels of sleep-inducing chemicals low. That's why any amount of caffeine consumption delays sleep onset (the time at night that you feel sleepy enough to nod off), reduces quality of sleep, and interferes with the stages of sleep, causing you to wake more often. Sleep researchers actually have an official phrase for it: caffeine-induced sleep disorder.

Now, here's the thing. Not everyone is sensitive to caffeine. Some people can drink a cup of coffee before bed and go right to sleep and not wake again until the alarm clock rings. Others drink a cup in the morning and are up all night. How do you know if you are caffeine sensitive? If you are a high-stress responder (type A), you probably can't have caffeine in the afternoon and still expect to get to sleep at night. Also, if you're the type of person who can give up coffee any given day and not notice an increase in fatigue or a headache, you're probably a low-caffeine responder.

To wean yourself off caffeine, keep track of how much of the stuff you drink and how often. Then, try to increase your caffeine-free hours before bed. For example, if you have your last cup of tea or coffee around 2 or 3 P.M., cut it back to 1 or 2 P.M. and then to noon. (Try replacing it with a power nap.)

Ask Pete

Q I just had a mole removed and now I can't sleep. What's going on?

A Whether you had a mole removed or laparoscopic surgery to take out your appendix, you need more sleep, and your body is going to resist you. A Danish study of twelve women shows that minor surgery (in this case a laparoscopic gallbladder removal) influenced the women's circadian rhythms, delaying the natural drop and rise in body temperature that signal sleep onset and wakefulness. Overcome this response with the thermostat advice at right.

PUT YOUR THERMOSTAT ON A TIMER: Sleep is induced, in part, by a drop in body temperature. A Japanese study of six women and two men determined that gradually decreasing nightly temperature from 80°F to 75°F at night and then increasing it from 75°F to 80°F in the morning helped trick the body into falling asleep more readily at night and waking with more alertness in the morning. You don't have to set your thermostat as high as the temperatures used in the study. The important point is to drop temperature by five degrees in the hour before bedtime and then set it to rise by five degrees in the hour before you want to wake up.

SLEEP ALONE ONCE OR TWICE A WEEK: Most people sleep more deeply when they are not sharing their bed with a partner or a pet. If your partner gets annoyed about you continually leaving your marriage bed, explain that the deeper sleep you get from sleeping alone will charge you up during the day, making you more receptive to his sexual advances. Trust me. I'm a guy. It works every time.

STAY UP LATER: If you suffer from insomnia, don't lie awake in bed. Doing so causes your brain to associate your bed with wakefulness. Use your bed for sleep and sex, and nothing else. If you do not fall asleep within thirty minutes of getting into bed, get up and go do something else. Stretch, read, or clean out a closet. Then try going back to bed. If you continually suffer from insomnia, stay up later and later until you feel so tired that you fall asleep as soon as your head hits the pillow. Then slowly increase your sleep time by going to bed a bit earlier each night.

Bottom Line: Whatever you do to improve sleep time and quality, keep it simple. Stressing yourself out by incorporating too many remedies at once will only make you toss and turn more. Try just one of my sleep solutions at a time, adding a new one every couple of weeks as needed.

MAKE HOUSE SPACE

It never ceases to amaze me how quickly a house, apartment, or computer can get filled up. I recently moved from a 1,200-square-foot apartment to a 5,000-square-foot home. I thought I'd have more space than I could ever need, but I expanded into my space. I bought furniture. I acquired things. I covered the walls with art and photographs.

As the stuff flowed in, I started to feel filled up. It made me feel heavy. The house was weighing on me. I realized that I had too much stuff. Now I take five minutes a few times a week to declutter. I might tackle a drawer, a closet, or a file cabinet. I find the space-finding mission cleansing and relaxing. It makes me feel lighter and freer.

If you are a die-hard organizer, my routine will seem second nature to you. If you are a stuff saver—and you know who you are—it will go against your grain. I encourage you to think about why you feel so attached to the clothes you haven't worn since the 1970s, your grown children's old bedroom furniture, and those shelves of novels that you've already read. I think you'll find the answer illuminating. By saving this stuff, you are trying to hold on to the past, but you just can't. Let the past go. It's gone anyway. Live in the present. Enjoy life now, and make space so you can enjoy it even more.

I encourage you to spend five minutes a few times a week at making space:

IN THE KITCHEN: Go through your pantry. Pull out all of the fake foods. Donate them to a food kitchen. Go to your spice rack. Get rid of any spice that's more than a year old. It's lost its kick, and it's preventing you from finding the spices you actually need. Do the same with old appliances. That bread maker? It's history.

IN YOUR CLOSET: Take out anything you haven't worn in the past year and donate it to charity. If you worry that you just might want to wear it again, put it in a box in your basement, attic, or garage. If after six months you haven't once thought about what you've stored in that big box, haul the box to Goodwill. Every time you buy new clothes that flatter your new body, get rid of an old outfit that you no longer wear.

IN YOUR DESK OR FILE CABINET: Take paper financial documents that you need for tax purposes, scan them into your computer, and then shred the paper. Use the shredded paper as packing material when you mail items. Do the same with paper photos. If they are not in an album or framed, scan them into your computer. Set the screen saver to show the photos, so you actually get to look at them every once in a while.

THROUGHOUT THE HOUSE: Walk through your house. Hang out in various rooms. Do any make you feel claustrophobic? Do you really need all of that furniture? Do you have chairs that you never sit in? Donate them to charity.

ON YOUR COMPUTER: Defragment your hard drive. Delete your cookies. Run the cleanup utility. Delete old e-mails and store the ones you need to save in individual folders.

IN YOUR CHECKBOOK: Sign up for automatic deductions for your mortgage, car payments, child care costs, life insurance, and any other bills that remain the same from month to month. It saves you time later on and eliminates those stressful moments when you realize you forgot to pay the mortgage. Plus it will earn you karma points. Experts estimate that for every 170 people who switch to auto deductions and e-banking, one tree is saved a year.

ON YOUR BOOKSHELF: Those books you haven't read in ten years? Donate them to the library so someone else can read them.

IN YOUR ENTERTAINMENT CENTER: Remove old games and movies that you no longer use or watch. Trade them in for something else. If you have kids, make a rule that no new game comes into the house until another one leaves.

IN YOUR KID'S TOY BOX: Continually sweep through it, removing anything your child hasn't played with in the past year. Make your child a part of this process. Allow your kid to choose the toy and, if possible, the younger child to hand it down to. Make a rule that for every new toy that comes into the house, an old toy must go out.

Bottom Line: Make your exercise days decluttering days. If you exercise seven days a week, then you declutter seven days a week. If you exercise three days a week, then you declutter three days a week.

PETE'S LIFE BALANCE SHEET

Keep track of your sleep, your stress level (using a 1-to-10 scale), your energy, and your mood on your scorecard. Whenever any of these dip below a 5 on the 1-to-10 scale, it's time to take a good hard look at your Life Balance Sheet. Your Life Balance Sheet is a "profit or loss" report that adds up your withdrawals (overworking yourself, overexercise, marital problems, etc.) and your deposits (your dedication to the 90-Second Fitness Solution, extra sleep, and incorporating the other advice in this chapter).

For good health, you want a balance with a surplus. If you allow your balance to dip below zero, you bounce a check. End result: you get sick. The more deposits you make, the greater your reserve and the more you can play hard without suffering undesirable consequences such as fatigue or anxiety.

I'm giving you 100 weekly "free" dollars. This is your salary. Each week, I'll deposit $100 into your account. You can add to that amount by making deposits (shown below), but you can also make withdrawals (shown below). The idea is to keep the account balanced.

ACTIVITY	DEPOSIT DOLLARS	WITHDRAWAL DOLLARS
One of Pete's workouts	10	
Running		20
Yoga	10	
Meditation or another relaxation technique	10	
Unaddressed marital issues		30
Great sex	15 (should be more)	
Late night of partying		20
Eating real food	10	
Eating fake food		10
Smoking		20
Each preschool-age child		20
Each school-age child		10
Each teenager		25

ACTIVITY	DEPOSIT DOLLARS	WITHDRAWAL DOLLARS
Supportive significant other who folds laundry and washes the dishes without being asked	15	
Supportive significant other who cooks dinner for you	400 (Priceless!)	
Unsupportive significant other who doesn't help, even when you ask for it		30
A recent bout of the cold or flu		30
Getting up earlier than usual		10
Staying up later than usual		10
Taking your supplements	10	
Being at your ideal body weight	10	
Being overweight		10
Listening to soothing music	10	
Getting a massage	15	
Laughing hysterically	15	
Snuggling with a loved one	10	
Snuggling with a loved one, getting turned on, and then having wild sex	35	
Petting a dog or cat	10	
Taking a vacation	10	
Taking a vacation without the family	100	
Sleeping in	10	
Sleeping in and then having morning sex	20	
Taking a power nap	10	

ACTIVITY	DEPOSIT DOLLARS	WITHDRAWAL DOLLARS
Taking a warm bath before bed	10	
Spending time in nature	10	
Reading a novel	10	
Not multitasking	5 (for each focused task)	
Multitasking		5 (for each unfocused task)
Quiet time	10	
Sleeping alone	15	
Decluttering your home	1 (for every minute spent doing it)	
Each year past your thirty-fifth birthday		1
Asking for help*	20	
A stressful job		40
Working overtime		10 (for every hour)
Taking Pete's supplements	10	

* If this were a book for men, asking for directions would be 100.

Got the idea? Let's take a typical week of one of my female clients, Alexis. She is forty-six years old, has a career (lawyer), a husband, and two kids. One child has problems in school, which causes Alexis to worry excessively and toss and turn at night. She's getting only five good hours of sleep each night. She doesn't eat well and takes no supplements, and before she met me she did no exercise at all. She's not overweight but has no muscle tone on her five-foot-four, 120-pound frame. She looks flabby even though she fits into a size four easily. Here are her withdrawals:

- 40 units for career
- 10 units for overtime
- 30 units for unhelpful husband
- 20 units (10 for each kid)
- 11 units for being 46 years old
- 20 units for poor sleep
- 10 units for poor diet

- 141 TOTAL

So our friend is using 141 units each week on a 100-unit budget. If this were money, she would be bankrupt. I told Alexis that she needed to make some deposits and perhaps stop making so many withdrawals. The fastest and easiest way to improve her score? Get rid of the husband and kids! She'd save 50 units! Problem solved. She'll live to see her hundredth birthday.

Okay, I was just kidding, although I know that solution is actually pretty tempting for some women, especially the idea of getting rid of the husband. It's not practical, though, and the divorce and custody issues would have probably cost her 65 units. Here is what I really did suggest.

Take power naps	10 units
Quiet time	10 units
Eat better	10 units
Take supplements	10 units
Pete's workout	10 units

Now our friend is working well within her budget and is able to cope with the weekly stress and any additional stresses that come her way.

WHAT'S NEXT?

You've just learned the fourth and last ingredient in the 90-Second Fitness Solution. You now have everything you need for total body health and fitness. If you haven't gotten started, I recommend you do so right now. Do a Wall Sit. Do the Plank. Go out and buy those supplements. Shop for real foods and clean the fake food out of your kitchen.

Turn the page to learn how to maintain your momentum and how to recommit yourself when you backslide. (And if you're thinking that *you* don't need to read chapter 6 because you won't backslide, you'd better turn the page if you know what's good for you.)

PART III

STRONG FOR LIFE

CHAPTER 6

Stay Successful

You might be wondering: Pete, look, if this is the most time-efficient plan ever, why in the world would I need advice to help me stick with it? If I can't maintain my results on this plan, what hope is there for me at all? First, there's hope. Lots of hope. Second, you need help because you are human. You are fallible. We all are. Even me.

Yes, even me, your faithful fitness crusader. Case in point: during the editing stages of this book, my coauthor asked me to review one of the chapters. I did it while holding my screaming eight-month-old. I sent it back to her, proud of myself for my ability to multitask. I soon got an e-mail with a series of questions about the chapter, about material I had no recollection reading. I opened the file and realized that I had only reviewed half of the chapter. I'd forgotten to read the second half. I'd also broken the very advice I'd suggested in that chapter. I'd multitasked to save time and I'd ended up wasting it instead.

Even I fall off my fitness and eating plans from time to time. Two things generally get me to miss workouts: poor eating and exhaustion, with one usually leading to the other. It usually goes like this. I go out on a Friday night and I give in to the hors

Backsliding is inevitable. We all do it, even me, and even Alisa. When you gain weight, stop exercising, forget your supplements, feel stressed out, and find yourself eating fast food, hot dogs, and Froot Loops, come to this chapter. Recommit by:

1. Forgiving yourself. You're human.
2. Making a New Year's resolution (no matter what day of the year it is) to get fit and healthy.
3. Putting on your bathing suit and training for bathing suit season.
4. Do the Wall Sit. Do the Plank—now!
5. Purchase any needed supplements.
6. Find and follow your perfect eating day. If you've gained weight, do a liquid diet, followed by an avocado-shake-salad diet, and *then* do the perfect eating days.
7. Spend fifteen minutes decluttering your home or office, and go to bed early.
8. Get up the next day and follow the 90-Second Fitness Solution as directed.

d'oeuvres and indulge in a martini. Once I get a buzz, I'm even more likely to eat the bread, rice, and other carbohydrate side dishes that accompany the main meal. When I weigh myself the next morning, I see that I'm a few pounds heavier. I'm also exhausted from getting in late the night before, so I rest and hit the cookies. They're my number-one comfort food.

Now it's Sunday. I sleep in, but I still wake groggy because I'm still tired from Friday night. Sunday is one of my scheduled workout days, but I blow off the workout because I'm in a coma and I can't snap out of it. I eat more refined carbs, particularly bread, cake, and cookies.

Then I weigh myself Monday morning. I'm now five pounds heavier. I'm disgusted with myself. I'm in a pissy mood because I missed my workout, and I feel like a BLIMP! See? It happens, even to me. I go through this scenario about three or four times a year. How come I haven't gained fifty pounds over the years? Because I know when to put an end to the backsliding and get myself recommitted to fitness.

When you backslide, come to this chapter. I don't care how often you have to come here. Come here every day for a month if needed. Just come here. When you stop taking your supplements, come here. When you can't button those jeans without sucking in your tummy, come here. When you buy that first bag of Cheez Doodles, come here. When you can't find your telephone because it's buried underneath your kid's toys, come here. When you haven't done the Plank in so long you think it's something you walk down, come here. Here I've provided you with my tried-and-true method for getting back on track. It's what works for me. It's what works for my clients and it will work for you.

GET BACK ON TRACK

Recommitting yourself starts with putting things in perspective. So what if you stopped strength training? Half of the people who start a new fitness plan—even one as short as this one—stop within the first six months. You're normal. So what if you drank too much wine or beer or had too many martinis or margaritas the night before and the night before that? It happens. So what if you ate way too much cake or pie or too many cookies over the holidays. Who doesn't? So what if you ran out of your supplements a few weeks ago and still have not gotten around to buying more? Alisa, my coauthor, goes through that scenario all the time. She orders her supplements online. Restocking her supply couldn't be easier or more convenient. Her favorite saying? "It's the things that take thirty seconds that I never get around to doing."

Yes, you've gained a few pounds. Yes, those dark circles are under your eyes yet again. Yes, you're tossing and turning at night. Yes, you feel groggy in the morn-

SUE LIEBMAN

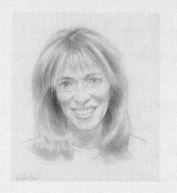

It was the spring before I turned forty. I'd had two kids, and after the second, I found myself with ten extra pounds that I couldn't seem to lose. A friend told me about Pete. I got his name and signed up. In addition to his workouts, I also changed what I ate. I stopped eating crap and started eating smart.

The results were dramatic. I lost ten pounds in just a couple of months, and then something amazing happened. I just kept losing. I was happy with losing just the ten pounds, but something about Pete's workouts made my body lose even more. I eventually plateaued at a twenty-five-pound weight loss. I dropped five clothing sizes. I now wear a size two. I'm smaller than I've ever been.

My body shape has changed too. I've always been the classic pear shape with the small upper body and the wide hips and thighs. The day I walked into the store, picked out a pair of slim-fit boys' jeans, slipped them on, and felt not one bit of tightness across my thighs was the most phenomenal day of my life. I thought: This can't be my body! I couldn't believe that I could actually wear jeans and look good in them too.

My husband has always been skinny and has always been really fit, but when he saw the changes in my body, he was curious. He started working out with Pete too. I must have sent Pete at least fifty other clients. People saw my results and wanted to know how I got them. I just told them what was true.

I've stuck with him for seven and a half years and have maintained my weight loss the entire time. When I tell people that I used to be twenty-five pounds heavier, they don't believe me. They look at me and marvel, "You're in such great shape." I always tell them that they can be too. They need only give Pete a call.

ing. Yes, you are reexperiencing the afternoon slump again. Yes, you feel like crap.

You know what? You already have the solution to these problems. It worked once, and it will work again. More important, it worked quickly. How hard was it to commit the first time? Not that hard, right? If I wanted you to do an hour-long workout that required you to change your clothes and take a shower afterward, I'd understand your reluctance to get back on track. If I wanted you to buy thirty different supplements every month, I could see how you might put off that trip to the health food store. If I wanted you to make gourmet meals every night, I could see how you'd continually blow it off. If I wanted you to spend thirty minutes relaxing every day, I could understand how that might stress you out.

I'm not asking for that much. This program is so simple that you can recommit anywhere and anytime, even in your office, in your hotel room, and at your kid's school.

You can recommit right now, this very moment, and you know what? You're going to come back better and stronger. We all make periodic pushes. No one trains consistently 365 days per year. We all ebb and flow. We all train and eat really well, slip up a little bit, recommit, and then train harder and better. Our progress resembles the up-and-down progress of the stock market. Yes, there are dips from time to time, and some of those dips are pretty dramatic, but over a period of years, there's an average 10 percent improvement. The same is true with your body. No matter how often, how long, or how dramatically you backslide, you are always better off than before you started this program. Got that?

Let's get started.

I'd like you to do a few things that will really fire up your commitment. First, I want you to pretend that today is January 2. I don't care if it's really May 20, July 4, or September 9. For you, it's January 2. It's time for a big push.

In my gym, January 2 marks the day we start training for swimsuit season. Go to your bedroom and find your swimsuit. Put it on. Yes, that's right, put it on, even if it's November and even if you never plan on wearing that particular suit again. Let's see what you look like. How ready is your body for swimsuit season? Not so ready? That's all the more reason to recommit.

Now, you can stay in your swimsuit or you can get dressed. It's your choice. For Step 2 in firing up your commitment, I want you to go back to your scorecards. Go get your

PDA, your notebook, or whatever it is that you used to keep track of your workouts, eating, and life. Go get it now. I'll wait.

Let's start with your fitness scorecard. Your notations will look something like this, depending on the workouts you were doing:

DATE	11/1	11/3	11/5	11/8	11/10	11/12	11/16
Wall Sit	62	68	71	77	80	88	90
Plank	34	45	51	55	63	67	72

(time in seconds)

See how well you were doing? You were kicking booty! See how strong you got and how quickly you got there? Do you see how you progressed from workout to workout? You were an animal. You can be that animal again. This scorecard will give you an idea of where to restart yourself.

> **IF YOU MISSED A WEEK:** Start with the previous workout. You probably haven't lost any strength. It takes a few weeks of missed workouts for strength to wither away.

> **IF YOU MISSED A MONTH:** Look at your scorecard to determine the rate of progress you can expect of yourself over a seven-workout period. Pick up right where you left off. The body doesn't lose strength as fast as everyone thinks. You'll be right back on top in a few workouts. I promise!

> **IF YOU'VE MISSED MORE THAN A MONTH:** Go back to step one, but be assured that you will fly through each level twice as fast. Muscles have memory. It doesn't take long to get back to where you were.

You've seen your results. Now I want you to do one better. Beat your own scorecard. Are you up to the challenge? Then put down the book, haul your butt out of the

La-Z-Boy, and go to the wall. That's right. You're recommitting and you are doing it this very minute. I don't care what workout you were doing before you stopped working out. This very moment you're doing the Wall Sit and the Plank. It's going to take you three minutes. You have three minutes, right? Just do it.

Still reading? Put down the book and get on the wall. Then get on the floor. Don't even think about coming back until you've done both.

I'm serious about this.

I really am.

Do I need to come to your house and haul you off the couch myself?

You're right. I really have no way of knowing whether or not you've followed Pete's orders, but I sure hope you have. Feel better? I bet you do. Starting over is cleansing. It boosts your confidence. You'll fly though the levels and goal times much more quickly than before and you'll get back to where you left off in no time.

Now let's talk about food. That's probably what got you into this health-related black hole in the first place. Take a look at your eating records on your scorecard. If you've been doing as I suggested in chapter 3, you've been writing down what you eat daily and you've also been keeping track of your weight, your energy level, your mood, or some other aspect of health that is important to you. Look at your records. Find a great day. Find a perfect day. Find a day that resulted in great ratings for weight, mood, energy, and whatever else you've been keeping track of. Find a day that you can easily re-create.

For example, in looking at my records, I realized that one morning I was four pounds lighter. I went back to my scorecard to see what I'd eaten the day before this dramatic weight loss. This is what it looked like:

7:00 A.M.   *100 percent organic carrot juice mixed with one scoop of whey protein powder, taken with supplements*

7:30 A.M.   *1 large cup of coffee with organic milk and organic sugar.* *

* This doesn't count as a meal, but my life doesn't start until I've had my coffee.

12:00 P.M.   *5 egg whites and a turkey burger with salsa*
              1 bottle of water

6:00 P.M.   *1 or 2 large avocados*

Have you found the perfect day? I'll wait. Go ahead and get those records.

Do we have to go through this again? Get off the couch and go find the records.

Okay, now here's what I'd like you to do. Use one of the following strategies, depending on the severity of your backsliding:

You haven't been eating as well as you'd like but you have not gained weight: Follow your perfect day of eating two days in a row. Then progress to the Real Food Diet.

You've gained three or more pounds: I say three pounds because anything less just might be water weight. Once you get to three, however, you need to break out of that water-weight denial and get serious about getting the scale to go in the opposite direction. If you've really strayed for a long time and have gained so much weight that you are thoroughly disgusted with yourself, then it's time for more drastic measures. Do the following:

1. Do my Liquid Diet (page 113) for twenty-four to forty-eight hours. Do it for twenty-four hours if you're only three pounds heavier. Do it for forty-eight if you've gained more than three pounds.
2. Follow the avocado-salad-shake diet (Step 2 of my Dress Diet plan outlined on pages 117 to 119) for twenty-four to forty-eight hours. Do it for twenty-four hours if you're only three pounds heavier. Do it for forty-eight if you've gained more than three pounds.
3. Follow your perfect eating day until you feel you've done the penance. That means you're back to your goal weight *and* you no longer feel guilty about your backsliding.

This three-step approach will kill those sugar cravings that have worked their way back into your life. It will also help you to reestablish a sense of control. It even punishes you a bit. Now you're going to associate falling off the plan with a negative consequence. It's just like the idea of your elementary school principal with the paddle. You may have never actually been smacked on the rear end with the paddle, but the idea of him having it kept you in line. The same goes for the three-step reinitiation. The idea of having to do it again will keep you on the straight and narrow.

So you've done your workout. You've got your eating under control. We still need to address two more aspects of the plan.

Let's talk about supplements. If you are out of supplements, get in the car, drive to the drug or health food store, and replenish your stash right now. Take them as directed.

Now let's talk about your life. You're grounded, okay. Your penance involves some clutter busting. Spend at least fifteen minutes organizing some part of your home or office. It might be a drawer, a cabinet, or a closet. I don't care what you organize. Just do it. Get a big box and toss any donatable items into it. Toss the rest into the recycling or the trash. Then, this evening I want you to take your 5-HTP and hit the sack early. I'm taking away your TV privileges. I don't want you to take part in any stimulating activity (with the exception of sex). Lights out at nine. Pete's orders.

HOW TO PREVENT BACKSLIDING

Now you're back. Let's keep you here.

The best way to avoid setbacks is to expect them. I've been training people for more than twenty years. During that time, I've developed a sixth sense about momentum and when they are going to lose it. I've learned that most people stray from the plan during one of the following times:

AUGUST: You'll go on vacation. Your vacation mind-set will tell you, "I'm on vacation. I can eat whatever I want." Your vacation mind-set will tell you, "I'm on vacation. I don't have access to a gym. I'll start working out again when I get home." You'll tell yourself, "I'm on vacation, I can stay out later and drink more alcohol than I do at home." And this is all true to some extent, as long as you don't mind being a couple pounds heavier at the end of your vacation.

The Solution: Stay on plan and still have a fantastic vacation. My mom and dad took the whole family on the *Queen Mary II* for a five-day cruise. I lost two pounds, and it wasn't from seasickness. I was there to relax. I wanted to catch up on some reading, go to the casino (my favorite), and hit the pool. When we sat down to all our meals, I chose a protein food and a vegetable. I indulged in a drink a day and I even hit the dessert bar. The extra walking (especially when we docked at a place with a beach) burned off the cookie and martini easily. Vacation is about rest and relaxation and fun, but it's not about getting as fat as you can. Go ahead and indulge a little more, but counteract that indulgence by walking more too. Also, there's no excuse not to get in your 90-Second Fitness workout. You have a wall and a floor. Use them.

HOLIDAYS: We all indulge a little, and in some cases a lot, on the holidays. That's what they are for.

The Solution: Before any big holiday meal, do your workout. It will put you in the right frame of mind. Start the meal with soup and salad, and put a heaping serving of steamed veggies on your plate. The soup, salad, and veggies will fill you up so you are less likely to overdo it on the mashed potatoes and cookies. Choose a protein food (turkey, chicken, fish) to go with your veggies, and you will be even less likely to inhale three slices of cake. Then take a walk after dinner to work off the pumpkin pie.

SOCIAL LIFE: Most of my clients can stick with their plan at home. It's when they go out with friends that everything seems to fall apart.

The Solution: Before you go out, have a protein shake. It will soothe your hunger, making you less likely to dive into the hard pretzels at the bar. While out, hold yourself to one alcoholic drink. To stick to just one, do one of two things. If you like beer, go for it. It takes a lot longer to drink a pint of beer than it does to drink a glass of wine, even though both contain similar amounts of alcohol and calories. Choose a hoppy beer such as an India Pale Ale (IPA) or any microbrew with a name like "Hops Explosion," "Hops Heaven," or "Double Hop." The bitterness of the hops will slow you down. If you prefer wine, choose a drier variety such as a cabernet or a chardonnay. Again, it's harder to toss back a dry wine than a fruity one, such as a pinot grigio. Have whatever you drink with a glass of water. Before you order a second drink, you must first down two glasses of club soda. The carbonation in the soda is going to slow you down and fill you up, making you less likely to order the second drink.

DISRUPTIONS: You're sick. Your kid is sick. You have to travel on business. You just got a promotion at work and you're really stressed about the new responsibilities. A family member is in hospice.

The Solution: Hey, it all happens. Don't stress yourself out when life gets overly stressful. Stick with basics. Return to the home workout. Stick with the Wall Sit and the Plank. You can do these anywhere, and they are great mood boosters and stress soothers. Reach for real foods as often as you can. Stick with the supplements and go easy on yourself.

HOW TO STAY MOTIVATED

Okay, you're back. You're psyched. Let's keep you here. Use the following advice:

WEIGH YOURSELF DAILY: According to the National Weight Control Registry, a study of thousands of people who had lost an average of sixty-six pounds and kept it off for five years found that dieters who are most likely to maintain their weight step on the scale daily. Weigh yourself at least five times per week, if not daily. If you're tempted not to weigh yourself on any given morning, examine that excuse. If I had a nickel for every client who pleaded, "Please don't weigh me this week," I would have a few bagfuls of nickels. It's on the days that you most don't want to weigh yourself that you probably most need to step on the scale. Your reluctance stems from your premonition that the number will be high. Just get on the scale. If it's more than two pounds above your idea, deal with it. Do my three-step weight-loss approach outlined in chapter 3, starting on page 112.

GO SHOPPING: There's nothing like a credit card bill to keep you on track. Buy your new stronger, tighter body lots of clothes. I'm talking Neiman Marcus clothes. I'm talking Ann Taylor. I'm talking J. Jill clothes. I'm talking "the-clothes-I-really-want-but-are-too-expensive" clothes. Once you buy them, you better make sure your body stays in shape while you pay off those credit cards. How? Simple. Stay on the plan.

WORK OUT FIRST, DO EVERYTHING ELSE SECOND: It's easy to think: "I'm busy, I'll do my workout later." Instead, I want you to think: "I'm busy, I'll do my workout now." If possible, do a workout on Monday mornings. I've noticed that most of my clients are more emotionally and physically rested on Mondays than they are on any other day of the week. They also have a lot of adrenaline in reserve, physical energy that they can pour into their workout. As the week progresses, however, problems at work or complications at home tend to burn people out, and their workouts become less effective and less enjoyable. When they switch to a Monday workout routine, they feel strong and confident all week long, which translates into more effectiveness at work and home.

CHALLENGE SOMEONE: Be boastful. Tell your teenage son or nephew, your spouse, your brother, or a friend that you're stronger than he or she is. Choose someone half your age or male. Choose someone who is going to say "Yeah right" when you make that "I'm stronger" statement. Put money on it. Create a huge wager. The loser has to clean the house, rub your feet, cook dinner, whatever. Make a wager that you'll really enjoy. Then challenge him to a Wall Sit or a Plank. Get on the wall or the floor and see who can hold the longest. I'm willing to bet that you're going to blow this poor guy's doors off. Of course he could do more reps than you. He can probably hoist more weight than you, but he probably doesn't have the endurance to last longer on the wall or in the plank. I know this because I've seen it time and time again. I've seen sixty-year-old women outlast thirty-year-old men. I've seen forty-five-year-old moms outlast their sixteen-year-old sons. There's nothing like the realization that you are stronger than a man or someone half your age to keep you motivated for more.

DO IT WITH YOUR SPOUSE, A FRIEND, OR YOUR KIDS: An exercise partner not only makes the workout seem more fun but he or she also can guilt you into doing it on those days when you'd like to tell yourself that you are too busy.

KEEP A SUPPLEMENT RESERVE ON HAND: Want to know why most people stop taking their supplements? They run out. As I've mentioned, this used to happen to my coauthor all of the time. Then she came up with this ingenious solution. She now buys two of everything. When she kicks the main bottle and starts on the spare, she writes "get multivitamin" on her to-do list.

KEEP SIMPLE STAPLES ON HAND: Simple staples are those foods you turn to at the end of the week when you've run out of groceries. They are the foods you eat when you are too tired to cook, and they are the foods I want you to turn to whenever you are craving fake food. Avocado, salsa, baby carrots, and cucumber, for example, all last a long time in the fridge and they all can be used for a quick real-food meal. Just smash up the avocado, mix it with the salsa, and dip the carrots and sliced cucumber in it. Voilà. You've got a real food meal in minutes, and it took less time than driving to the closest fast food restaurant. Here are some staples to keep on hand at all times:

› Whey protein for shakes.

› Avocados.

> › Hard-boiled eggs.

> › Cans of water-packed tuna and wild salmon.

> › Nuts and seeds.

> › Olives, especially the more flavorful varieties such as kalamata.

> › Ricotta cheese.

> › Bell pepper, cucumber, baby carrots, and any other veggies that you like to eat raw.

CREATE EASY WEEKS: We all get busy from time to time. We all celebrate holidays, travel, and otherwise find ourselves with weeks from hell. When that happens, I want you to use home workout Level 1, page 35. Don't feel guilty about this. If you can't get to the gym, you can't get to the gym, but you can do something, and home workout Level 1 is it.

KEEP THE FAITH: The longer you follow the plan and the more often you recommit, the better your long-term success. It's just like any habit. It's hardest in the beginning. The more you get yourself back on track, the less often you will fall off the wagon in the future, and the more easily you'll climb back on once you fall off.

WHERE TO GO FROM HERE

Some fitness professionals will have you believe that you need to continually make progress to improve or maintain your body. They'll tell you to push, push, push. Once you can sit on the wall for 90, these folks tell you to go for 100 and then 150. They tell you to get your butt to the gym and go heavy, heavier, and heavier still.

By now, you've probably got an inkling that I'm a little different from most of the fitness professionals you might meet, and this idea of continual progression is no different. Every time I get into a debate with these misguided wannabes, I always turn the tables on them and ask, "So you must be lifting about nine hundred pounds yourself by now, right?" Blank stare. Humans are not designed to make continual progress indefinitely.

So get yourself into a comfortable rhythm. Get to your goal weight. Get to a place where you feel good—you're energetic, happy, and confident. Get to good health.

And then stay there. There's no need to push any further than what I've laid out for you. You don't have to kill yourself to look and feel good. Look at all the people who are eating six times a day, doing endless aerobics, changing their workout routines constantly, and taking $600 worth of supplements each month. Do they look better than you? Are they happier? Do they have more energy?

Nope, nope, and nope.

Keep it simple. In life there are some things that are essential and some things that are elective. My plan gives you everything that is essential and nothing that's elective. You can tackle the electives if you want, but always remember that they are not requirements. In the end, staying fit and healthy comes down to this: life is short—get away with everything you can! You've built a beautiful body and a beautiful life, and you should feel damn proud of yourself.

CHAPTER 7

Recipes and Resources

In the following pages, I've provided you with everything you need to follow my Real Food Diet. It's my hope that the recipes and recommended products, will keep you on track for months and years to come. It's not necessary for you to use only these recipes and only the products I've recommended. They are here to help you keep things simple. Use what works best for you.

SIMPLE RECIPES

In the following pages, you'll find thirty-three recipes. Many come straight from my or my coauthor's recipe file. A few were donated by my clients. Some were developed by Jennifer Kushnier, a chef and friend, and Leslie Dantchik, a nutrition expert and colleague. All of the recipes are simple and:

1. Require very little cleanup. Most of them use just one pot, and in some cases, easy cleanup is worked into the cooking method.

2. Call for only a few ingredients, and 99 percent of those ingredients are available at any major grocery store. No specialty-store shopping is required.

3. Need very little prep time. Although some of the following recipes may take as long as thirty minutes to cook, most take only five minutes or fewer to prepare. Many can be eaten raw; they're perfect for women who use their ovens as storage space.

4. Use very little in the way of appliances. If you have a knife, a mixing bowl, a casserole dish, a blender and/or a food processor, a microwave, and an oven, you can make all of these recipes.

5. Do not require you to know much about cooking. If you can chop vegetables and turn on your oven or microwave, you can make these recipes.

These recipes also incorporate my Real Food Diet rules. You'll find very little in the way of flour products, processed ingredients, and dairy. My first priority in creating a recipe, however, is flavor. If eliminating the cheese, dairy, or another borderline ingredient results in mush that even my coauthor's dog doesn't want to eat, it's just not worth it. For that reason, I've included a few borderline foods in some of the recipes. Eating real isn't an all-or-nothing proposition. You can make conscious decisions. If you eat real most of the time, you'll have a little room for half-and-half, cheese, and even whole wheat pasta.

Enjoy!

BREAKFAST DISHES

90-SECOND MOCHA CAPPUCCINO

My day does not start until I have my coffee. Why not get my caffeine fix with my morning shake?

- 1 bottle Bolthouse Farms Perfectly Protein Mocha Cappuccino
- 1 scoop whey protein

Place in a blender or shaker bottle and blend until smooth.

Serves 1.

90-SECOND RICOTTA

When you're on the go and feeling just a little decadent, turn to this morning option. Yes, ricotta is a borderline food, but if it keeps you away from the doughnuts, then it's done its job.

- $\frac{1}{4}$ to $\frac{1}{2}$ cup part-skim ricotta
- 1 tablespoon ground flaxseeds or flax meal
- 1 scoop whey protein
- $\frac{1}{4}$ cup sliced fruit

Place ricotta, flax, and whey protein in a small bowl. Mix thoroughly with a fork. Gently combine with sliced fruit.

Serves 1.

GARDEN OMELET

This omelet is loaded with vegetables, but there's no need to slow yourself down by pulling out the measuring spoons and cups. Omelets are forgiving. Just eyeball your ingredients, putting as many veggies in the omelet as you can fit.

6 whole eggs,* whipped

$\frac{1}{4}$ cup spinach, chopped

3 tablespoons canned chopped tomatoes, drained

$\frac{1}{4}$ cup bell pepper, chopped

1 tablespoon yellow onion, chopped

1 tablespoon canned black beans, rinsed and drained

1 cooked turkey sausage link, sliced

Heat a large oiled skillet over medium-low heat. Add eggs. Sprinkle spinach over the egg, then add the tomatoes, pepper, onion, beans, and sausage. Once bottom and edges are cooked through, slide a spatula under the omelet and flip one side over the other. Remove from heat, slice into two crescents, and serve.

Serves 2.

Use 1 whole egg and 6 whites if you're trying to lose weight.

GINGER VEGETABLE SHAKE

This drink is a great way to get in a vegetable serving. The ginger adds some zip to it. If it's too spicy for you, just leave out the ginger.

1 bottle Bolthouse Farms Vedge (vegetable juice)

1 scoop whey protein

Pinch of fresh ginger, peeled and chopped

Place in a blender and process until smooth.

Serves 1.

JENNIFER'S FRITTATA ITALIANA

You probably don't have time to bake a frittata during the work week, so make a couple of pans on a Sunday. Wrap the leftovers in plastic wrap. It will keep for up to three days. If paired with a bowl of fresh fruit or 1 or 2 slices of turkey bacon, this recipe can stretch to 4 servings. Simple tip: Instead of opening an entire jar or can, get your pepper and artichoke hearts from your supermarket's salad bar.

5 softened sundried tomatoes, cut into quarters (about 1 tablespoon)

4 eggs, 8 egg whites, or 1 cup liquid egg product

1 tablespoon light cream

$\frac{1}{8}$ teaspoon salt and a couple of grinds of fresh pepper

$\frac{1}{2}$ teaspoon dried basil

2 to 3 artichoke hearts in water, chopped (about 3 tablespoons)

$\frac{1}{2}$ roasted red pepper, roughly chopped (about 2 tablespoons)

$\frac{1}{2}$ teaspoons minced fresh or jarred garlic

$\frac{1}{2}$ tablespoon olive oil

2 tablespoons freshly grated or shredded Parmesan cheese

Fill a small bowl with hot water. Place tomatoes in the bowl to reconstitute, about 10 minutes. Preheat the oven to 350°F. Set one rack in the middle of the oven and one rack beneath the broiler.

In a bowl, whisk the eggs until frothy. Add the cream, salt, pepper, and basil. Whisk again. Add the vegetables to the eggs and stir gently.

Heat the olive oil in an 8-inch oven-safe skillet over medium heat until hot, swirling the pan to coat the bottom with oil, about 1 minute. Pour the egg mixture onto the hot skillet. Bake on the middle rack until the eggs set, about 12 minutes. Remove the skillet from the oven and top with the cheese. Put the pan under the broiler until the cheese melts and browns slightly, about 2 minutes. Remove from the oven and remove the frittata from the pan. Loosen the edges, and it should lift right out.

Serves 2.

JENNIFER'S SAVORY WINTERTIME FRITTATA

Make a couple of frittatas on a Sunday. Wrap the leftovers in plastic wrap. It will keep for up to three days. If paired with a bowl of fresh fruit or 1 or 2 slices of turkey bacon, this recipe can stretch to 4 servings.

$\frac{1}{2}$ tablespoon olive oil

1 tablespoon shallot, minced

4 cremini ("baby bella") mushrooms, sliced thin

$\frac{1}{4}$ teaspoon fresh thyme

4 eggs, 8 egg whites, or 1 cup liquid egg product

1 tablespoon light cream

$\frac{1}{8}$ teaspoon salt and a couple of grinds of fresh pepper

$\frac{1}{2}$ tablespoon olive oil

2 tablespoons grated or shredded Parmesan cheese
(not the dry canned cheese!)

Preheat oven to 350°F. Set one rack in the middle of the oven and one rack beneath the broiler. Heat the olive oil in an 8-inch oven-safe skillet over medium-low heat. Add the shallots, mushrooms, and thyme. Cook, stirring occasionally, until the mushrooms are soft and the shallots translucent, about 5 to 6 minutes. Remove from heat and cool slightly.

In a small bowl, whisk the eggs until frothy. Add the cream, salt, and pepper. Whisk again.

Add the cooled mushroom-shallot mixture to the eggs and stir gently.

Wipe the skillet with a paper towel and add the second $\frac{1}{2}$ tablespoon oil. Heat over medium heat until hot, swirling the pan to coat the bottom with oil, about 1 minute. Pour the egg mixture into the hot skillet and bake on the middle rack until the eggs set, about 10 minutes. Remove the pan from the oven and top with the cheese. Put the pan under the broiler until the cheese melts and browns slightly, about 2 minutes. Remove from the oven and remove the frittata from the pan. Loosen the edges, and it should lift right out.

Serves 2.

JENNIFER'S SMOKED SALMON FRITTATA

Make a couple of frittatas on a Sunday. Wrap the leftovers in plastic wrap. It will keep for up to three days. If paired with a bowl of fresh fruit or 1 or 2 slices of turkey bacon, this recipe can stretch to 4 servings.

4 eggs, 8 egg whites, or 1 cup liquid egg product

1 tablespoon light cream

$\frac{1}{8}$ teaspoon salt and a couple of grinds of fresh pepper

1 teaspoon chopped chives

$\frac{1}{4}$ cup smoked salmon, pulled apart into small pieces and
    picked over for any tiny bones

1 tablespoon capers, drained (optional)

$\frac{1}{2}$ tablespoon olive oil

Light sour cream

Preheat the oven to 350°F. Set a rack in the middle of the oven.

In a small bowl, whisk the eggs until frothy. And the cream, salt, pepper, and chives. Whisk again. Add the salmon and optional capers and stir gently.

Heat the olive oil in an 8-inch oven-safe skillet over medium heat until hot, swirling the pan to coat the bottom with oil, about 1 minute. Pour the egg mixture into the hot skillet and then bake until the eggs set, about 12 minutes. Remove from the oven. Remove the frittata from the pan. Loosen the edges, and it should lift right out. Serve with a dollop of sour cream if desired.

Serves 2.

LESLIE'S STRAWBERRY-BANANA SMOOTHIE

If you're the type of person who has irregular bowel habits (you know who you are), the flax in this drink will get you regular.

- 1 cup frozen organic whole strawberries, unsweetened
- 1 medium banana
- $\frac{1}{2}$ cup plain fat-free yogurt (organic, preferred)
- 2 tablespoons organic ground flaxseed
- 1 teaspoon honey

Place in a blender and process until smooth.

Serves 1.

NICHOLAS'S APPLE-BANANA SHAKE

My oldest son, Nicholas, turned me on to this shake. We were walking through the streets of Manhattan and stopped by a fresh juice stand located outside a restaurant. It was 4 P.M., and we were due for a snack. As we looked down the menu, Nicholas pointed out the apple, banana, and cinnamon combo. I said, "All we need is a scoop of whey protein and this would be perfect!" The juice stand had GNC Whey Protein. We ordered two.

- 8 ounces water
- 1 apple, peeled and cored
- 1 banana
- 1 scoop whey protein
- 1 teaspoon cinnamon
- 3 ice cubes

Place in a blender or shake bottle and blend until smooth.

Serves 1.

STRAWBERRY PROTEIN SMOOTHIE

Don't ask me why, but I lean toward this one on cold or rainy days. Maybe it's a pick-me-up that I don't know about. Either way, it gets me off to a good start.

$\frac{1}{2}$ cup plain fat-free yogurt (organic, preferred)

1 scoop whey protein

1 cup frozen organic whole strawberries, unsweetened

Place in a blender and process until smooth.

Serves 1.

MAIN DISHES

90-SECOND GUACAMOLE

If you don't have a lot of time to slice and dice, try this simple guacamole version. When my coauthor offered it to her husband, he asked, "Wow, how did you make this?" It tasted so gourmet that he was stunned that she'd created it simply by mixing together two ingredients.

> 1 avocado, sliced, pitted, and mashed
> 1 to 2 tablespoons salsa

Mix avocado with salsa and serve. Eat plain with a spoon or use as a dip for baby carrots, celery, or other vegetables. You can also spoon it onto romaine hearts and enjoy as a "sandwich."

Serves 1.

ALISA'S FAVORITE ONE-POT MEAL

Alisa created this recipe when she was experimenting with poached chicken. She had a lot of broth left over and wanted to put it to good use. Voilà, the next time she made Simplest Ever Poached Chicken (page 194), she added the couscous and spinach, creating a complete one-pot meal. In lieu of spinach, you may use any favorite green, such as mustard greens, collards, or chard. To simplify cooking, don't bother to measure the spinach. Just add as much to the pan as you can fit!

> 1 tablespoon cooking oil
> $\frac{1}{2}$ onion, diced
> 1 to 2 cloves garlic, chopped

1½ pounds chicken breast, boneless and skinless

2 cups chicken stock

2 to 3 tablespoons curry powder or cumin

1 11-ounce box whole wheat couscous*

2 to 3 cups baby spinach, densely packed

Heat oil in a large skillet over medium heat. Add onion and garlic. Cook for about 3 minutes until onions are translucent. Add chicken, chicken stock, and curry. Bring to a simmer and then reduce heat to low, cooking for 15 minutes. Do not allow to boil. Add couscous, stirring it into the broth. Cook for 5 minutes, and then add spinach. Once spinach wilts and chicken is completely cooked through, serve.

Serves 4.

In lieu of whole wheat couscous, you can also use decoated quinoa (nearly all quinoa sold in North America is already decoated). Quinoa is a true power food that is rich in protein, minerals, and fiber. Add the quinoa after cooking the chicken for 10 minutes. Then simmer for 10 minutes before adding the spinach.

ALISA'S FAVORITE STUFFED PEPPERS

I got Alisa hooked on avocados soon after we started working together, and soon after she began putting them in everything. Even so, the following recipe seemed like green eggs and ham to her. She was fairly certain that she'd end up tossing the whole thing in the trash the first time she made it. Then she tried the concoction, and now it's one of her family's favorites.

1 avocado, pitted and skinned

3 tablespoons chopped red onion

1 tablespoon canned black beans, rinsed and drained

2 tablespoons canned diced tomato, drained

Juice of ½ lime

1 cup lump crabmeat (optional)

1 bell pepper, halved lengthwise and seeded

2 to 3 tablespoons shredded cheese

Place avocado in a small bowl. Mash with a fork. Combine with onion, beans, tomatoes, lime juice, and optional crabmeat. Spoon into the pepper halves. Sprinkle cheese on top. Cook in the microwave for 2 minutes, or for 20 minutes in a 375°F preheated oven, until cheese melts and pepper is warm but still crisp.

Serves 2.

HUMONGOUS SALAD

Enjoy this salad for lunch or dinner during the Skinny Black Dress Diet.

1 to 2 cups lettuce, spinach, or any dark green leafy vegetable

1 to 2 cups chopped vegetables (broccoli, cauliflower, cucumber,
    bell pepper, etc.)

3 ounces salmon or skinless chicken or turkey breast or 1 to 2
    hard boiled eggs

2 tablespoons balsamic vinegar

1 tablespoon olive oil

Lemon juice, salt, and pepper to taste

Cover a large plate with the greens and top with the vegetables and meat or eggs. Toss with vinegar, olive oil, lemon juice, salt, and pepper.

Serves 1.

JENNIFER'S CALI BURGER

I bet you didn't think you'd ever mix avocado into a hamburger, now did you? Not only does it add healthful fats and fiber, but the avocado also keeps it moist.

$\frac{1}{4}$ clove garlic

$\frac{1}{4}$ avocado, peeled and pitted

$\frac{1}{2}$ teaspoon lime juice

$\frac{1}{4}$ teaspoon dried cumin

A couple of grinds of pepper and a good pinch of salt

$\frac{1}{4}$ of a 1.3-pound package 99 percent lean ground turkey

$\frac{1}{2}$ teaspoon Worchestershire sauce (optional)

Olive oil

Sliced red onion

Sliced tomato

Optional: guacamole, salsa, or $\frac{1}{2}$ whole wheat bun

Mince garlic in a food processor. Add avocado and lime juice and process until finely minced. Transfer avocado mixture to a small bowl and mash further with a fork or the back of a spoon. Add spices. Break apart the turkey with your hands and add to the bowl along with the Worchestershire sauce. Mix it all together with your fingers, squishing it to blend the avocado with the turkey.

Form a patty. If any avocado bits fall off the burger, press them back in. With turkey, a wide and thin patty is better than a short and fat one. The patty should be less than 1 inch thick. Create a small well in the center by using your thumb to make a slight indentation.

Lay foil on a baking sheet and oil lightly. Lay the burger on the oiled foil (indented side facing up) and place under the broiler for 5 minutes. Flip and cook for another 5 minutes. Turn off the broiler and allow the burger to rest in the oven while you prepare your fixings. Serve topped with onion and tomato. Add guacamole or salsa or eat open-faced on a whole wheat bun.

Serves 1.

JENNIFER'S EASTERN BURGER

This turkey burger is loaded with fiber, thanks to the wheat germ. Consider eating it and other burgers Pete's way, with a knife and fork. This eliminates the need for a bun and allows you to pile all sorts of interesting veggies on top.

- 2 teaspoons olive oil
- 1 tablespoon minced shallot (roughly $\frac{1}{2}$ to 1 whole shallot)
- $\frac{1}{2}$ teaspoon garlic (roughly $\frac{1}{2}$ clove)
- 2 tablespoons chopped cremini ("baby bella") mushrooms, either 1 large or 2 small, roughly chopped into small pieces
- Salt and pepper to taste
- 1 tablespoon low-sodium soy sauce
- $\frac{1}{2}$ teaspoon brown rice vinegar
- $\frac{1}{2}$ teaspoon chili paste
- $\frac{1}{4}$ of a 1.3-pound package 99 percent lean ground turkey
- 1 tablespoon raw wheat germ
- Chopped scallion, both green and white parts
- Optional: guacamole, sliced avocado, sliced veggies
- $\frac{1}{2}$ whole wheat bun

Heat the oil in a pan over medium heat. Add the shallot and the garlic and cook until just sizzling, stirring occasionally. Add the mushrooms, stir, and add salt and pepper. Cook until just starting to brown. Add the soy sauce, vinegar, and chili paste. Stir to combine, then remove pan from heat. Cool slightly.

Break apart the turkey with your hands and add to a small bowl along with the wheat germ. Mix together. Add mushroom mixture to turkey mixture, combining it with your fingers, squishing it to blend the mushrooms with the turkey.

Form a patty. If any veggie bits fall off the burger, simply press them back in. With turkey, a wide and thin patty is better than a short and fat one. The patty should be less than 1 inch thick. Create a small well in the center by using your thumb to make a slight indentation.

Lay foil on a baking sheet and oil lightly. Lay the burger on the oiled foil (indented side facing up) and place under the broiler for 5 minutes. Flip and cook for another 5 minutes. Turn off the broiler and allow the burger to rest in the oven while you prepare the burger fixings. Top with scallions, guacamole, sliced avocado, or your favorite sliced veggies. Eat open-faced on a whole wheat bun.

Serves 1.

JENNIFER'S FISH TACOS

Fish tacos provide a delicious way to sneak in a number of vegetables, as the following recipe shows. No bread crumbs? No problem! Simply put any nonsweet crackers into a Ziploc bag, crush, then roll them with a rolling pin until pulverized.

$\frac{1}{2}$ pound filet of fish such as turbot, flounder, halibut, or sole, cut in half

1 tablespoon flour

5 tablespoons unseasoned bread crumbs or panko (Japanese bread crumbs)

1 tablespoon butter

1 tablespoon olive oil

1 egg, beaten

Dash of salt and pepper

Two 8- or 10-inch whole wheat or spinach tortillas

$\frac{1}{4}$ cup grated cheddar cheese (or Mexican/taco cheese blend)

$\frac{1}{4}$ cup chopped tomato

$\frac{1}{4}$ cup chopped green cabbage or lettuce of choice

2 tablespoons red or Spanish onion, chopped

$\frac{1}{4}$ cup diced avocado

Juice of half a lime

Rinse and pat the fish dry.

Spread the flour and the bread crumbs on separate plates.

Heat the butter and the oil in a medium frying pan over medium heat until melted. Swirl the pan to combine them and cover the bottom of the pan.

Pat both sides of the fish into the flour, covering all the flesh. Then dredge each filet in the egg. Next, lay each filet in the bread crumbs, covering both sides of the fish completely.

Lay each filet in the heated pan, sprinkle with salt and pepper, and cook for 4 to 5 minutes until golden. Flip the filets and cook 3 to 4 minutes more. The fish is done when it flakes when forked. Remove pan from heat.

Lay each filet on its own tortilla. Divide the remaining ingredients, except the lime juice. Sprinkle each filet with cheese, tomatoes, cabbage or lettuce, onion, and avocado. Drizzle with lime juice. Roll up the tortilla and enjoy.
Serves 2.

JENNIFER'S STUFFED PEPPERS

To seed a pepper, use Jennifer's simple seeding technique: cut around the top of it, as if you were carving a pumpkin. Gently pull out the seed cluster. If the seed cluster won't budge, just lop off the entire top of the pepper. You don't need it.

1 red, orange, or yellow pepper (it should be shaped
   so it can stand upright), seeded
1 cup cooked wild rice, prepared according to package directions
   but with vegetable or chicken broth instead of water
$\frac{1}{2}$ cup canned salmon, pulled apart into small pieces and
   picked over for any tiny bones

¼ cup dried cranberries

Salt and pepper to taste

⅛ teaspoon dried sage

¼ cup chopped cremini ("baby bella") mushrooms

Preheat the oven to 350°F. Put the pepper standing upright in a small baking dish filled with ¼ inch of water. Bake uncovered until crisp-tender, about 15 minutes. For a softer pepper cook up to 30 minutes but don't allow it to scorch. Remove from the oven.

When the rice is done, add the salmon, cranberries, salt and pepper, sage, and mushrooms to the rice in the pot. (This simplifies cleanup.) Stir until combined.

Press the mixture into the pepper. The amount of filling could easily fill two peppers, or you can really stuff it into and mound it over one, but there will still be some left over for a tasty snack with crackers. Return the pepper to the oven and heat through, about 10 minutes.

Serves 1.

Variation:

1 cup cooked whole-grain couscous, prepared according to package
directions but with vegetable or chicken broth instead of water, and no butter

½ cup canned salmon, pulled apart into small pieces and picked
over for any tiny bones

¼ cup dried cranberries

4 teaspoons chopped scallions (green and white parts)

Salt and pepper, to taste

Assemble according to the main recipe instructions.

JOLYNN'S AS REAL AS IT GETS PASTA

You've probably never considered putting beets, pumpkin seeds, or feta cheese in your pasta sauce. Neither had we. When Jolynn gave us this recipe to include in the book, Alisa and I discussed, "How are we going to tell her that we can't use it? This can't possibly taste good." Then Alisa brazenly made the recipe one night when she had vegetarian dinner guests. Everyone raved about it! It was the best pasta sauce they'd ever tasted.

Good thing too, because beets and beet greens are among nature's superfoods, providing plenty of antioxidants, folic acid, potassium, iron, and calcium. To simplify cooking, roast beets once a week. Wash the beets thoroughly. (Save the greens. You'll need them for the recipe.) Slice off the tops. Cover a casserole dish with parchment paper (to simplify cleanup). Place beets on the paper, tightly cover with foil, and bake for 30 to 60 minutes at 425°F until a fork can easily pierce them. Remove and cool. Slide off the skins. Store in a bag in the fridge until use.

1 tablespoon cooking oil

$\frac{1}{2}$ yellow onion, chopped

2 cloves garlic, chopped

2 golden beets,* roasted (see top note for roasting instructions) and chopped

Greens from two beets, deveined and steamed

$1\frac{1}{2}$ cups cremini "baby bella" mushrooms

2 cups pasta sauce (see list of recommended brands on page 204)

14.5-ounce box whole-grain pasta, cooked according to package instructions

Pumpkin seeds to taste

Crumbled feta cheese to taste

Heat oil in a skillet over medium heat. Add onions and garlic. Cook for 3 to 5 minutes, until onions are translucent. Add beets, beet greens, and mushrooms. Cook for 5 minutes, until mushrooms are warm and soft. Add sauce. Reduce heat to low. Cook pasta for 5 more minutes until sauce is heated through.

Serve over pasta. Top with pumpkin seeds and feta cheese.

Serves 6

If you can't find golden beets, use red beets. They lend a similar flavor but will turn your sauce a bright cranberry red.

LESLIE'S SUPER SPICY SHRIMP TACOS WITH BLACK BEANS AND BROWN RICE

These tacos provide everything you need. No side dishes required!

1½ tablespoons olive oil, divided

1 medium onion, sliced

1 clove garlic, chopped

2 cups sliced red, yellow, and green peppers

½ small jalapeño, chopped

½ tablespoon chili powder

½ tablespoon ground cumin

Sea salt and pepper to taste

½ pound medium shrimp (approx. 15–18), cleaned and deveined,
   tails removed

2 8-inch whole wheat soft tortillas

½ cup tomato salsa, divided

Optional: 1 tablespoon chopped cilantro

For extra spicy: add dash of hot sauce

For less spicy: leave out jalapeño and adjust seasoning to taste

Heat a medium skillet on medium to high heat for 1 minute. Add 1 tablespoon of the olive oil and coat the pan. Add onion. Cook until onions are translucent and soft (about 3 to 4 minutes). Add garlic, peppers, jalapeño, chili powder, cumin, salt, pepper, and $\frac{1}{2}$ tablespoon more olive oil, stirring constantly until mixture is complete coated. When peppers soften, toss in shrimp and cook until pink and opaque (approximately 1 to 2 minutes).

Cut tortillas in half and place on plates. Heat in microwave for 15 seconds to warm. Spoon mixture on top, add 1 to 2 tablespoons to each taco wrap, and enjoy. Serve with $\frac{1}{4}$ cup black beans and $\frac{1}{4}$ cup cooked brown rice on the side.
Serves 2.

MARYLOU'S CHICKEN SOUP

I'm especially proud of this recipe because it came from one of my favorite women on the planet, my mom. Plus, it doesn't get any simpler than this. Even my ten-year-old son can make this soup.

   32-ounce carton chicken broth
   1 bag frozen vegetables, any variety
   1 whole precooked chicken, meat carved and removed from the bone

Place all ingredients in a medium pot. Bring to a boil. Reduce heat to low. Simmer for 5 minutes and then serve.
Serves 4.

PETE'S FAVORITE GUACAMOLE

I usually eat guacamole plain with a spoon. You can also use this recipe as a dip for baby carrots, celery, or other vegetables. You can also spoon it onto romaine hearts and enjoy it as a "sandwich."

   1 to 2 whole avocados*
   $\frac{1}{2}$ teaspoon salt

3 tablespoons chopped onions

1 teaspoon chopped jalapeño

1 teaspoon chopped fresh or dried cilantro

1 chopped tomato (discard the juice and seeds) or $\frac{1}{3}$ 15-ounce
   can chopped tomatoes, drained

1 tablespoon lemon juice

Mash the avocados and mix with remaining ingredients.

Serves 1.

Simple Smarts: The fastest and easiest way to peel an avocado is by cutting it in half and squeezing the skin, as if you're squeezing the juice from a lemon.

SIMPLEST EVER AVOCADO SOUP

This soup is deceptively filling. It's a complete meal by itself and will stave off dessert cravings for days.

1 serrano pepper (or jalapeño if more heat is desired)

1 small clove garlic

1 tablespoon packed cilantro leaves*

1 small avocado

$1\frac{1}{4}$ teaspoons lime juice

1 cup vegetable or chicken broth

Dash of salt and a couple of grinds of fresh pepper

$\frac{1}{8}$ teaspoon chili powder

1 tablespoon light sour cream or Greek-style yogurt

2 tablespoons chopped cooked shrimp or small cocktail shrimp

Cut the pepper in half lengthwise, then in half lengthwise again. Remove the vein of seeds and cut the quarter-pepper in half crosswise. Peel the clove of garlic and cut it in half. Cut it in half again. Put the pepper and garlic into the bowl of a food processor and process until roughly chopped. Add the cilantro to the food processor and process until blended. Cut the avocado in half, squeeze the flesh from the two halves into the food processor, and process until smooth and creamy. Add the lime juice and the broth, $\frac{1}{3}$ cup at a time, and process until combined. (If the bowl of your food processor isn't large enough, add as much of the broth as you can, then add the rest after the next step.)

Pour the contents of the food processor into a small saucepan. Add the spices and stir to combine. Cook over low heat until heated through. Do not boil. Serve with a dollop of sour cream or Greek-style yogurt and top with the shrimp.
Serves 2.

*Simple Smarts: Because the stems of cilantro are quite tender, save time by using them intact. There's no need to pick the leaves off the stems.

SIMPLEST EVER POACHED CHICKEN

Poaching is the simplest, most healthful, and most delicious way to cook meat or fish. It's simple because the moistness of the cooking method prevents ingredients from sticking to the pan and necessitating an elbow grease–intensive cleanup. It's healthful because the water prevents toxins called advanced glycation end products (AGEs) from proliferating during cooking. Dry-heat cooking methods—baking, broiling, grilling, and microwaving—all increase these toxins. Finally, the liquid keeps the meat so tender that you don't even need a knife as you eat.

1 tablespoon cooking oil
$\frac{1}{2}$ onion, diced
1 to 2 cloves garlic, chopped
$1\frac{1}{2}$ pounds chicken breast, boneless and skinless
2 cups chicken stock
2 to 3 tablespoons curry powder or cumin

Heat oil in a large skillet over medium heat. Add onion and garlic. Cook for about 3 minutes until onions are translucent. Add chicken, stock, and curry. Bring to a simmer, then reduce heat to low, cooking for 15 to 20 minutes until chicken cooks through. Do not allow to boil. Serve plain, with extra curry powder to taste, or topped with Alisa's Favorite Tapenade, page 199, 90-Second Salsa, page 198, or guacamole.

Serves 3 to 4.

SIMPLEST EVER POACHED SALMON

Baking and other dry-heat methods can easily dry out fish. Let's keep it simple. Just poach it. Even if you overcook the salmon, you won't ruin it. It will still taste tender and juicy.

4 cups stock, chicken or vegetable

$\frac{1}{2}$ cup dry white wine (such as chardonnay)

2 pounds wild salmon

Bring stock and wine to a boil over high heat. Add salmon and reduce heat to medium-low, cover and cook for about 10 minutes until salmon is cooked through. Serve plain or topped with 90-Second Salsa, page 198, Alisa's Favorite Tapenade, page 199, or guacamole.

Serves 4.

SIMPLEST EVER POACHED SALMON: ALMOST-AS-SIMPLE VARIATION

For a little extra flavor and a gourmet touch, try this slightly more involved salmon recipe.

1 tablespoon cooking oil

$\frac{1}{3}$ cup red onion, chopped

$\frac{1}{3}$ cup celery, chopped

$\frac{1}{3}$ cup carrots, chopped

1 clove garlic, chopped

4 cups stock, chicken or vegetable

$\frac{1}{2}$ cup dry white wine (such as chardonnay)

2 pounds wild salmon

Heat oil in a stockpot over medium-high heat. Add onion, celery, carrots, and garlic. Cook for about 5 minutes until onions are translucent. Add stock and wine. Increase heat to high. Bring to a boil. Add salmon and reduce heat to medium-low, cover, and cook for about 10 minutes until salmon is cooked through. Serve plain or topped with 90-Second Salsa, page 198, Alisa's Favorite Tapenade, page 199, or guacamole. *Serves 4.*

TUNA GARDEN SALAD

Most people make sandwiches out of tuna salad, but this healthier version helps you optimize those vegetable servings.

Unlimited salad greens and chopped vegetables of your choice

$\frac{1}{2}$ avocado, sliced

3 ounces water-packed chunk light tuna or canned wild salmon

1 tablespoon olive oil

1 tablespoon chopped celery

1 tablespoon chopped onion

Dash of lemon juice

Lettuce

Cover a large dinner plate with salad greens, chopped vegetables of your choice, and sliced avocado. In a small bowl, mix tuna with olive oil, celery, onion, and lemon juice. Place tuna mixture over lettuce.

Serves 1.

SIDE DISHES, APPETIZERS, TOPPINGS, AND SNACKS

90-SECOND SALSA

When you're entertaining guests, use this incredibly quick topping to give chicken or fish a gourmet taste. They'll never guess that it took you a minute or two to throw together.

- 1 cup fresh pineapple, chopped
- 1 banana, chopped
- $\frac{1}{3}$ small red onion, chopped
- 2 tablespoons lemon juice

Combine all ingredients in a small bowl. Serve over fish or chicken.
Serves 4.

90-SECOND TRAIL MIX

For the healthiest trail mix, use only unsweetened and unsulphured fruits and unsalted and raw nuts. Most health food stores and many high-end grocery stores have self-serve bins where you can take as much or as little as you need.

- $\frac{1}{3}$ cup banana chips
- $\frac{1}{2}$ cup dried apricots
- $\frac{1}{4}$ cup dried currants (or wild blueberries)
- $\frac{1}{4}$ cup dried cherries (or raisins or cranberries)
- $\frac{1}{3}$ cup dried pineapple pieces
- 10 dried apples rings, broken in half
- $\frac{1}{4}$ cup almonds
- $\frac{1}{4}$ cup cashews

FROZEN FOODS

Amy's Brown Rice and Veggies Bowl

Amy's Indian Mattar Paneer

Amy's Indian Palak Paneer

Amy's Indian Vegetable Korma

Amy's Mexican Casserole Bowl

Amy's Teriyaki Bowl

Dr. Praeger's California Veggie Balls

Dr. Praeger's Spinach Littles

Kashi Black Bean Mango

Kashi Chicken Florentine

Kashi Lemon Rosemary Chicken

Kashi Lemongrass Coconut Chicken

Kashi Lime Cilantro Shrimp

Kashi Southwest-Style Chicken

Kashi Sweet and Sour Chicken

Simply Organic Beef Casserole

Simply Organic Beef Chili Con Carne

Simply Organic Chicken & Chickpea Korma

Simply Organic Lamb Tagine

Simply Organic Lentil and Vegetable Stew

Simply Organic Mixed Bean Chili

Simply Organic Moroccan Tagine

Simply Organic Roasted Vegetables with Quinoa

Simply Organic Thai Vegetable Curry

Simply Organic Vegetable and Bean Casserole

CANNED AND JARRED FOODS

Amy's Fire Roasted Vegetable Salsa

Amy's Medium Chili

Amy's Organic Alphabet Soup

Amy's Organic Black Bean & Corn Salsa

Amy's Organic Chili

Amy's Organic Chunky Tomato Bisque

Amy's Organic Chunky Vegetable Soup

Amy's Organic Family Pasta Sauce

Amy's Organic Fire Roasted Southwestern Vegetable Soup

Amy's Organic Garlic Mushroom Pasta Sauce

Amy's Organic Lentil Soup

Amy's Organic Lentil Vegetable Soup

Amy's Organic Medium Chili with Vegetables

Amy's Organic Medium Salsa

Amy's Organic Mild Salsa

Amy's Organic Roasted Garlic Pasta Sauce

Amy's Organic Spicy Chipotle Salsa

Amy's Organic Tomato Basil Pasta Sauce

Amy's Puttanesca Sauce

Amy's Refried Beans with Green Chilis

Amy's Refried Black Beans

Annie's Naturals BBQ sauces

Annie's Naturals Ketchup

Annie's Naturals mustard, any variety

Annie's Naturals salad dressings

Drew's Salsa

Dr. Pete's Chipotle Grilling Sauce

Enrico's pasta sauces, salsas, and black bean dip

Francesco Rinaldi Organic Roasted Garlic Pasta Sauce

Fresh Market Tomatillo Green Chili Salsa

Green Mountain Gringo Salsa, any flavor

Healthy Valley Minestrone

Healthy Valley Split Pea (no salt added)

Healthy Valley Vegetarian Bean Chili (no salt added)

Nellie and Joe's Key West Style Mojo Criollo

Newman's Own Organic Chunky Medium Salsa

Newman's Own Organic Cilantro Medium Salsa

Newman's Own Sweet Onion and Roasted Garlic Pasta Sauce

Progresso Healthy Classics Lentil

Salpica salsa

Seeds of Change Indian Simmer Sauce, any flavor

Seeds of Change Pasta Sauce, any flavor

Seeds of Change salad dressings

Silver Palate salsa

Simply Organic soup, any variety

Smart Balance Omega peanut butter

Texas Trading Company salsa

Worthington Low Fat Chili

DAIRY

Organic Valley cheese and yogurt

SHAKE MIXES

Bolthouse Farms Vedge
Bolthouse Farms Perfectly Protein Mocha Cappuccino
Odwalla Carrot Juice
Odwalla Superfood

SUPPLEMENTS

Carlson Fish Oil
http://www.carlsonlabs.com

GNC
www.gnc.com

Jarrow Formulas
http://www.jarrow.com

Nature Made
http://www.naturemade.com

Nordic Naturals
http://www.nordicnaturals.com

Solgar
http://www.solgar.com

YOUR 90-SECOND SCORECARDS

I've included all of your scorecards here for convenience. Photocopy the scorecard that corresponds to the workout you are using, and fill it in every day to keep track of your success on the 90-Second Fitness Solution. Alternatively, you can download and print out these scorecards from www.90secondfitnesssolution.com or create your own and keep track of this information using a PDA, cell phone, or laptop.

HOME WORKOUT #1

Date: _____   Weight: _____

WHAT I ATE

Breakfast

Lunch

Dinner

☐ Multivitamin   ☐ Fish Oil   ☐ 5-HTP

☐ Vitamin C   ☐ B Complex

ENERGY	1	2	3	4	5	6	7	8	9	10
MOOD	1	2	3	4	5	6	7	8	9	10
STRESS	1	2	3	4	5	6	7	8	9	10

DO I WANT TO NAP?

Morning   Y   N

Midmorning   Y   N

Midafternoon   Y   N

MOVEMENT	TIME IN SECONDS
1. Wall Sit	
2. Plank	

HOME WORKOUT #2

Date: _____   Weight: _____

WHAT I ATE

Breakfast

Lunch

Dinner

☐ Multivitamin   ☐ Fish Oil   ☐ 5-HTP

☐ Vitamin C   ☐ B Complex

ENERGY	1	2	3	4	5	6	7	8	9	10
MOOD	1	2	3	4	5	6	7	8	9	10
STRESS	1	2	3	4	5	6	7	8	9	10

DO I WANT TO NAP?

Morning	Y	N
Midmorning	Y	N
Midafternoon	Y	N

MOVEMENT	TIME IN SECONDS
1. Superwoman	
2. Wall Sit	
3. Leg Raise	
4. Sit-up	
5. Hangin' Out	
6. Plank	

HOME WORKOUT #3

Date: _____   Weight: _____

WHAT I ATE

Breakfast

Lunch

Dinner

☐ Multivitamin   ☐ Fish Oil   ☐ 5-HTP

☐ Vitamin C   ☐ B Complex

ENERGY	1	2	3	4	5	6	7	8	9	10
MOOD	1	2	3	4	5	6	7	8	9	10
STRESS	1	2	3	4	5	6	7	8	9	10

DO I WANT TO NAP?

Morning	Y	N
Midmorning	Y	N
Midafternoon	Y	N

MOVEMENT	TIME IN SECONDS
1. Superwoman	
2. Wall Sit	
3. Hindu Squat	
4. Leg Raise	
5. Sit-up	
6. Reverse Pull-up	
7. Push-up	

GYM SCORECARD

Date: _____   Weight: _____

WHAT I ATE

Breakfast

Lunch

Dinner

_____

☐ Multivitamin   ☐ Fish Oil   ☐ 5-HTP

☐ Vitamin C   ☐ B Complex

_____

ENERGY	1	2	3	4	5	6	7	8	9	10
MOOD	1	2	3	4	5	6	7	8	9	10
STRESS	1	2	3	4	5	6	7	8	9	10

_____

DO I WANT TO NAP?

Morning   Y   N

Midmorning   Y   N

Midafternoon   Y   N

_____

Movement	WEIGHT	TIME	REPS	OPTION	NEXT WEIGHT
Abduction machine					
Lower-back machine					
Leg press					
Rotary torso machine					
Abdominal machine					
Row					
Shoulder press					

90-second scorecard

ACKNOWLEDGMENTS

The Beginning

I would never have found the courage to stand up for the ideas that eventually became this book had the following people not supported me, continually encouraging me to better myself and my career. I especially thank my family: my sons, Nicholas and Jack; my mom, Marylou; my dad, Pete Sr.; my brother, Steve, and his family—Tito, Anthony, and Gabriella. Your love and support give me the strength to reach for what I would otherwise consider unattainable.

Thank you Aimée Bell for being "Patient Zero." We fondly call you that because it all started with you. Thank you for your enthusiasm and belief in something different.

Rae Krelitz: We're approaching twenty years of me torturing you and you putting up with me. Thank you for patiently watching me develop into the person I am today. Thanks also for your love and support. It defies the test of time.

I have been told that I have changed many people's lives, but Ruth Pomerance changed mine. Thank you, Ruth, for your support, friendship, and generosity. It opened many doors for me, and all of the amazing people who made this book a reality can be traced back to you.

What good is a good idea if no one knows about it? Thank you, Sue Liebman, aka "Susie Muscles," for telling everyone about me, my program, and my book. You trusted me to get you in shape, and I trusted you to be my orthodontist. It seemed fair, even though you had the ability to cause more pain. Maybe I should have had you tighten my braces *before* I made your arms so strong?

My Dream Team

I knew my program worked. I knew it was effective and simple. I believed in it with all my heart, but believing in something doesn't get it on a bookshelf. This program would never have gotten recorded onto the pieces of paper between these two covers had it not been for the following people.

David Vigliano of Vigliano Associates: Thank you for accepting this challenge and for representing me. For as long as I can remember, I've been pushing people to do better. Thank you for pushing me to do better.

Mike Harriot of Vigliano Associates: Thank you for one of the greatest e-mails I've ever received, titled "Great News." Thank you for coming to my gym and experiencing the program, just so you could better represent this project. Your guidance has been phenomenal.

Judith Curr, executive vice president and publisher of Atria Books: Thank you for taking a chance and believing in me not only as an author but also as your trainer. You've enriched my life.

Nick Simonds, my editor at Atria Books: Thank you for coming in to see the program firsthand before making your decision. Your guidance from blank page to published book cannot be measured.

Alisa Bowman: They say things happen in threes. For me this is true as far as this book is concerned. David and Mike agreed to represent me. Judith and Nick agreed to publish my book, and when I thought it couldn't get any better, you agreed to write it with me. Thank you for revisiting strength training with an open mind and embracing this program. I must have had the look of a proud parent the day you told me you could do a pull-up. Thank you for making this a great experience.

My Support System

David, Mike, Judith, Nick, and Alisa were the dream team, but the following people all played important supporting roles.

Mike Austin: Don't mix business with friendship? Nonsense! You've been my friend for well over ten years, and I wouldn't want anyone else as a business partner. Thanks for spreading the word in Pennsylvania as well as finding simple solutions to complex problems. Thanks for helping me develop the program and design the equipment.

Karen Kuchar: Thank you for bringing my exercises to life with your talented illustrations. You got down on the floor and got on the wall, just to make sure you drew the exercises correctly. You made my day when you told me that the Wall Sit and the push-up were the most challenging exercises you've ever tried. Thanks for living the program that you drew.

Jennifer Kushnier, Leslie Dantchik, Marylou Cerqua (aka Mom), Jolynn Baca, and Carol Staubi: No program is complete without great food. Thank your for designing some of the simple yet amazing recipes in this book.

Jolynn Baca, Sue Liebman, Sheila Hanna, Wendy Cohen, Karen Mann, Veronica Weismann, Cynthia Mann Haiken, Michele Kaplan, Carol Staubi, Julie Siegel, and Sara Wilford: Thank you for sharing your stories and being a part of this book.

Essential Exercise: Thank you, Todd Hudson and Mary Beth Holland, for considering something out of the ordinary and embracing it. Thank you for believing in my program and making it a success with your professionalism.

Rita Rivest: They say "out of sight, out of mind." Not true. Your name comes up often, even though you are on the West Coast. Thank you for believing in me from three thousand miles away.

Mike Ferretta: I remember you asking me at your London Court home, "Have you started any businesses this year?" That was 1984. Well, to say the least we have started a few over the last twenty-four years! From South Shore Muscles & Fitness to Chrono-DynaMetrics to this very book, you were there every step of the way. Thank you for your guidance and friendship. It's great to know that you are just a phone call away.

Anton Thompson: Over the years, we have often commented about the genetically gifted. Well, with twenty-five years in this profession, I've never met a trainer more gifted than you. Your personality, knowledge, and instincts are unmatched. Only a real friend would indulge me when I go off the deep end with new ideas. Thanks for being there every step of the way. Thanks for letting me bounce ideas off you and for your honest opinions. And by the way, your 7:30 A.M. is here waiting for you.

Bonnie Ammer: Thank you for your support and guidance throughout this process. Your enthusiasm for my program and belief in me will not go unnoticed. No. This does not mean I will be nice to you during your workout.

Twenty-four-hour support: Thank you, Lauren Albert, Melissa Austin, Sue Reed, Christine Reichle, and Nicole Schaffer for being an e-mail or phone call away whenever I needed anything. Friends like you kept me moving forward when things felt immovable.

Thank you to all my clients. Over the years I have learned something from each and every one of you. Thank you for choosing me when so many choices were available.

A special thank-you to my favorite client, Matt Haiken. I look forward to discussing the book in detail with you.

—Pete Cerqua

Mike Harriot: I will forever remember the day you called and suggested I hire you to be my agent. If it weren't for you, I'm sure I'd be locked away in a mental institution, spending my days banging my head against the wall. Thank you for removing me from the rat race and helping me to envision a more fulfilling career. Nick Simonds: Thanks for catching all of my mathematical errors, helping us to refine the manuscript, and ever so patiently explaining how to get the exercise illustrations placed on the right pages. Mark and Kaarina: Thank you for allowing me to type late at night, on the weekends, and in my sleep. I love you both more than I will ever be able to describe. You are my sunshine, my rainbows, and my rocks. Pete: Thank you for getting my body stronger and tighter in less time than it takes me to shower. I hated strength training until I met you. Now I think of you whenever I do a pull-up. Where were you when I was in eighth grade and couldn't climb the ropes in gym class?

—Alisa Bowman

SELECTED BIBLIOGRAPHY

CHAPTER 1

Cauza E, Hanusch-Enserer U, Strasser B, Ludvik B, Metz-Schimmerl S, Pacini G, Wagner O, Georg P, Prager R, Kostner K, Dunky A, Haber P. "The relative benefits of endurance and strength training on the metabolic factors and muscle function of people with type 2 diabetes mellitus," *Archives of Physical Medicine and Rehabilitation*. 2005 Aug; 86(8):1527–33.

Delagardelle C, Feiereisen P, Autier P, Shita R, Krecke R, Beissel J. "Strength/endurance training versus endurance training in congestive heart failure," *Medicine and Science in Sports and Exercise*. 2002 Dec; 34(12):1868–72.

Edworthy J, Waring H. "The effects of music tempo and loudness level on treadmill exercise," *Ergonomics*. 2006 Dec 15; 49(15):1597–610.

Izquierdo M, Ibanez J, Gonzalez-Badillo JJ, Hakkinen K, Ratamess NA, Kraemer WJ, French DN, Eslava J, Altadill A, Asiain X, Gorostiaga EM. "Differential effects of strength training leading to failure versus not to failure on hormonal responses, strength, and muscle power gains," *Journal of Applied Physiology*. 2006 May; 100(5):1647–56. Epub 2006 Jan 12.

Izquierdo M, Ibanez J, Hakkinen K, Kraemer WJ, Larrion JL, Gorostiaga EM. "Once weekly combined resistance and cardiovascular training in healthy older men," *Medicine and Science in Sports and Exercise*. 2004 Mar; 36(3):435–43.

Kraemer WJ, Ratamess NA. "Hormonal responses and adaptations to resistance exercise and training," *Sports Medicine*. 2005; 35(4):339–61.

Linnamo V, Pakarinen A, Komi PV, Kraemer WJ, Hakkinen K. "Acute hormonal responses to submaximal and maximal heavy resistance and explosive exercises in men and women," *Journal of Strength and Conditioning Research*. 2005 Aug; 19(3):566–71.

Macone D, Baldari C, Zelli A, Guidetti L. "Music and physical activity in psychological well-being," *Perceptual and Motor Skills.* 2006 Aug; 103(1):285–95.

Narloch JA, Brandstater ME. "Influence of breathing technique on arterial blood pressure during heavy weight lifting," *Archives of Physical Medicine and Rehabilitation.* 1995 May; 76(5):457–62.

Pierson LM, Herbert WG, Norton HJ, Kiebzak GM, Griffith P, Fedor JM, Ramp WK, Cook JW. "Effects of combined aerobic and resistance training versus aerobic training alone in cardiac rehabilitation," *Journal of Cardiopulmonary Rehabilitation.* 2001 Mar-Apr; 21(2):101–10.

Rubin MR, Kraemer WJ, Maresh CM, Volek JS, Ratamess NA, Vanheest JL, Silvestre R, French DN, Sharman MJ, Judelson DA, Gomez AL, Vescovi JD, Hymer WC. "High-affinity growth hormone binding protein and acute heavy resistance exercise," *Medicine and Science in Sports and Exercise.* 2005 Mar; 37(3):395–403.

Schmitz KH, Ahmed RL, Yee D. "Effects of a 9-month strength training intervention on insulin, insulin-like growth factor (IGF)-I, IGF-binding protein (IGFBP)-1, and IGFBP-3 in 30-50-year-old women," *Cancer Epidemiology, Biomarkers and Prevention.* 2002 Dec; 11(12):1597–604.

Singh NA, Clements KM, Fiatarone MA. "A randomized controlled trial of progressive resistance training in depressed elders," *Journals of Gerontology.* Series A, *Biological Sciences and Medical Sciences.* 1997 Jan; 52(1):M27–35.

Smutok MA, Reece C, Kokkinos PF, Farmer C, Dawson P, Shulman R, DeVane-Bell J, Patterson J, Charabogos C, Goldberg AP. "Aerobic versus strength training for risk factor intervention in middle-aged men at high risk for coronary heart disease," *Metabolism: Clinical and Experimental.* 1993 Feb; 42(2):177–84.

Szabo A, Small A, Leigh M. "The effects of slow- and fast-rhythm classical music on progressive cycling to voluntary physical exhaustion," *Journal of Sports Medicine and Physical Fitness.* 1999 Sep; 39(3):220–5.

Westcott WL, La Rosa Loud R, Cleggett E, Glover S. "Effects of regular and slow speed training on muscle strength," *Journal of Sports Medicine and Physical Fitness.* 2001 Jun; 41(2):154–8.

Westcott WL, La Rosa Loud R, Glover S. Strength training frequency. Unpublished study available at http://www.ssymca.org/quincy/westcott/research_studies.htm.

Yamashita S, Iwai K, Akimoto T, Sugawara J, Kono I. "Effects of music during exercise on RPE, heart rate and the autonomic nervous system," *Journal of Sports Medicine and Physical Fitness*. 2006 Sep; 46(3):425–30.

CHAPTER 2

Askling C, Karlsson J, Thorstensson A. "Hamstring injury occurrence in elite soccer players after preseason strength training with eccentric overload," *Scandinavian Journal of Medicine Science and Sports*. 2003 Aug; 13(4):244–50.

Audette JF, Jin YS, Newcomer R, Stein L, Duncan G, Frontera WR. "Tai chi versus brisk walking in elderly women," *Age and Ageing*. 2006 Jul; 35(4):388–93. Epub 2006 Apr 19.

Barnett A. "Using recovery modalities between training sessions in elite athletes: Does it help?" *Sports Medicine*. 2006; 36(9):781–96.

Beneka A, Malliou P, Fatouros I, Jamurtas A, Gioftsidou A, Godolias G, Taxildaris K. "Resistance training effects on muscular strength of elderly are related to intensity and gender," *Journal of Science and Medicine in Sport*. 2005 Sep; 8(3):274–83.

Carpinelli RN, Otto RM. "Strength training. Single versus multiple sets," *Sports Medicine*. 1998 Aug; 26(2):73–84.

Cauza E, Hanusch-Enserer U, Strasser B, Ludvik B, Metz-Schimmerl S, Pacini G, Wagner O, Georg P, Prager R, Kostner K, Dunky A, Haber P. "The relative benefits of endurance and strength training on the metabolic factors and muscle function of people with type 2 diabetes mellitus," *Archives of Physical Medicine and Rehabilitation*. 2005 Aug; 86(8):1527–33.

Christou M, Smilios I, Sotiropoulos K, Volaklis K, Pilianidis T, Tokmakidis SP. "Effects of resistance training on the physical capacities of adolescent soccer players," *Journal of Strength Conditioning Research*. 2006 Nov; 20(4):783–91.

Davis J, Murphy M, Trinick T, Duly E, Nevill A, Davison G. "Acute effects of walking on inflammatory and cardiovascular risk in sedentary post-menopausal women," *Journal of Sports Science*. 2007 Oct 17; 1–7. Epub ahead of print.

Delagardelle C, Feiereisen P, Autier P, Shita R, Krecke R, Beissel J. "Strength/endurance training versus endurance training in congestive heart failure," *Medicine and Science in Sports and Exercise*. 2002 Dec; 34(12):1868–72.

DiFrancisco-Donoghue J, Werner W, Douris PC. "Comparison of once-weekly and twice-weekly strength training in older adults," *British Journal of Sports Medicine*. 2007 Jan; 41(1):19–22. Epub 2006 Oct 24.

Fatouros IG, Kambas A, Katrabasas I, Leontsini D, Chatzinikolaou A, Jamurtas AZ, Douroudos I, Aggelousis N, Taxildaris K. "Resistance training and detraining effects on flexibility performance in the elderly are intensity-dependent," *Journal of Strength Conditioning Research*. 2006 Aug; 20(3):634–42.

Fatouros IG, Taxildaris K, Tokmakidis SP, Kalapotharakos V, Aggelousis N, Athanasopoulos S, Zeeris I, Katrabasas I. "The effects of strength training, cardiovascular training and their combination on flexibility of inactive older adults," *International Journal of Sports Medicine*. 2002 Feb; 23(2):112–9.

Fletcher IM, Anness R. "The acute effects of combined static and dynamic stretch protocols on fifty-meter sprint performance in track-and-field athletes," *Journal of Strength Conditioning Research*. 2007 Aug; 21(3):784–7.

Galvão DA, Taaffe DR. "Resistance exercise dosage in older adults: Single- versus multiset effects on physical performance and body composition," *Journal of the American Geriatric Society*. 2005 Dec; 53(12):2090–7.

Herbert RD, de Noronha M. "Stretching to prevent or reduce muscle soreness after exercise," *Cochrane Database of Systematic Reviews* (online). 2007 Oct 17; (4):CD004577.

Herbert RD, Gabriel M. "Effects of stretching before and after exercising on muscle soreness and risk of injury: Systematic review," *British Medical Journal*. 2002 Aug 31; 325(7362):468.

Jones AM. "Running economy is negatively related to sit-and-reach test performance in international-standard distance runners," *International Journal of Sports Medicine*. 2002 Jan; 23(1):40–3.

Liu-Ambrose T, Khan KM, Eng JJ, Janssen PA, Lord SR, McKay HA. "Resistance and agility training reduce fall risk in women aged 75 to 85 with low bone mass: A 6-month randomized, controlled trial," *Journal of the American Geriatric Society.* 2004 May; 52(5):657–65.

Li Y, McClure PW, Pratt N. "The effect of hamstring muscle stretching on standing posture and on lumbar and hip motions during forward bending," *Physical Therapy.* 1996 Aug; 76(8):836–45; discussion 845–9.

Mikesky AE, Mazzuca SA, Brandt KD, Perkins SM, Damush T, Lane KA. "Effects of strength training on the incidence and progression of knee osteoarthritis," *Arthritis and Rheumatism.* 2006 Oct 15; 55(5):690–9.

Peate WF, Bates G, Lunda K, Francis S, Bellamy K. "Core strength: A new model for injury prediction and prevention," *Journal of Occupational Medicine and Toxicology.* 2007 Apr 11; 2:3.

Pierson LM, Herbert WG, Norton HJ, Kiebzak GM, Griffith P, Fedor JM, Ramp WK, Cook JW. "Effects of combined aerobic and resistance training versus aerobic training alone in cardiac rehabilitation," *Journal of Cardiopulmonary Rehabilitation.* 2001 Mar-Apr; 21(2):101–10.

Schmitz KH, Ahmed RL, Yee D. "Effects of a 9-month strength training intervention on insulin, insulin-like growth factor (IGF)-I, IGF-binding protein (IGFBP)-1, and IGFBP-3 in 30-50-year-old women," *Cancer Epidemiology Biomarkers and Prevention.* 2002 Dec; 11(12):1597–604.

Shrier I. "Does stretching improve performance? A systematic and critical review of the literature," *Clinical Journal of Sports Medicine.* 2004 Sep; 14(5):267–73.

Singh NA, Clements KM, Fiatarone MA. "A randomized controlled trial of progressive resistance training in depressed elders," *Journals of Gerontology. Series A, Biological Sciences and Medical Sciences.* 1997 Jan; 52(1):M27–35.

Smutok MA, Reece C, Kokkinos PF, Farmer C, Dawson P, Shulman R, DeVane-Bell J, Patterson J, Charabogos C, Goldberg AP, et al. "Aerobic versus strength training for risk factor intervention in middle-aged men at high risk for coronary heart disease," *Metabolism: Clinical and Experimental.* 1993 Feb; 42(2):177–84.

Stewart LK, Flynn MG, Campbell WW, Craig BA, Robinson JP, Timmerman KL, McFarlin BK, Coen PM, Talbert E. "The influence of exercise training on inflammatory cytokines and C-reactive protein," *Medicine and Science in Sports and Exercise*. 2007 Oct; 39(10):1714–9.

Stewart KJ, McFarland LD, Weinhofer JJ, Cottrell E, Brown CS, Shapiro EP. "Safety and efficacy of weight training soon after acute myocardial infarction," *Journal of Cardiopulmonary Rehabilitation*. 1998 Jan-Feb; 18(1):37–44.

CHAPTER 3

Adebamowo CA, Cho E, Sampson L, Katan MB, Spiegelman D, Willett WC, Holmes MD. "Dietary flavonols and flavonol-rich foods intake and the risk of breast cancer," *International Journal of Cancer*. 2005 Apr 20; 114(4):628–33.

Adebamowo CA, Spiegelman D, Berkey CS, Danby FW, Rockett HH, Colditz GA, Willett WC, Holmes MD. "Milk consumption and acne in adolescent girls," *Dermatology Online Journal*. 2006 May 30; 12(4):1.

Adebamowo CA, Spiegelman D, Danby FW, Frazier AL, Willett WC, Holmes MD. "High school dietary dairy intake and teenage acne," *Journal of the American Academy of Dermatology*. 2005 Feb; 52(2):207–14.

Anderson JW, Hoie LH. "Weight loss and lipid changes with low-energy diets: comparator study of milk-based versus soy-based liquid meal replacement interventions," *Journal of the American College of Nutrition*. 2005 Jun; 24(3):210–6.

Bandera EV, Kushi LH, Moore DF, Gifkins DM, McCullough ML. "Consumption of animal foods and endometrial cancer risk: A systematic literature review and meta-analysis," *Cancer Causes and Control*. 2007 Nov; 18(9):967–88. Epub 2007 Jul 19.

Bello NT, Hajnal A. "Male rats show an indifference-avoidance response for increasing concentrations of the artificial sweetener sucralose," *Nutrition Research*. 2005 Jul; 25(7):693–9.

Bergstrom BP, Cummings DR, Skaggs TA. "Aspartame decreases evoked extracellular dopamine levels in the rat brain: An in vivo voltammetry study," *Neuropharmacology*. 2007 Dec; 53(8):967–74. Epub 2007 Sep 29.

Berkey CS, Rockett HR, Willett WC, Colditz GA. "Milk, dairy fat, dietary calcium, and weight gain: A longitudinal study of adolescents," *Archives of Pediatrics and Adolescent Medicine*. 2005 Jun; 159(6):543–50.

Bigal ME, Krymchantowski AV. "Migraine triggered by sucralose—a case report," *Headache*. 2006 Mar; 46(3):515–7.

Bryner RW, Ullrich IH, Sauers J, Donley D, Hornsby G, Kolar M, Yeater R. "Effects of resistance vs. aerobic training combined with an 800 calorie liquid diet on lean body mass and resting metabolic rate," *Journal of the American College Nutrition*. 1999 Apr; 18(2):115–21.

Bulló M, Casas-Agustench P, Amigó-Correig P, Aranceta J, Salas-Salvadó J. "Inflammation, obesity and comorbidities: The role of diet," *Public Health Nutrition*. 2007 Oct; 10(10A):1164–72.

Chan P, Tomlinson B, Chen YJ, Liu JC, Hsieh MH, Cheng JT. "A double-blind placebo-controlled study of the effectiveness and tolerability of oral stevioside in human hypertension," *British Journal of Clinical Pharmacology*. 2000 Sep; 50(3):215–20.

Chang JC, Wu MC, Liu IM, Cheng JT. "Increase of insulin sensitivity by stevioside in fructose-rich chow-fed rats," *Hormone and Metabolic Research*. 2005 Oct; 37(10): 610–6.

Chavarro JE, Rich-Edwards JW, Rosner B, Willett WC. "A prospective study of dairy foods intake and anovulatory infertility," *Human Reproduction* (Oxford, England). 2007 May; 22(5):1340–7. Epub 2007 Feb 28.

———. "A prospective study of dietary carbohydrate quantity and quality in relation to risk of ovulatory infertility," *European Journal of Clinical Nutrition*. 2007 Sep. 19. Epub ahead of print.

———. "Dietary fatty acid intakes and the risk of ovulatory infertility," *American Journal of Clinical Nutrition*. 2007 Jan; 85(1):231–7.

Chiu HF, Tsai SS, Yang CY. "Nitrate in drinking water and risk of death from bladder cancer: An ecological case-control study in Taiwan," *Journal of Toxicology and Environmental Health* Part A. 2007 Jun; 70(12):1000–4.

Chiuve SE, Giovannucci EL, Hankinson SE, Zeisel SH, Dougherty LW, Willett WC, Rimm EB. "The association between betaine and choline intakes and the plasma concentrations of homocysteine in women," *American Journal of Clinical Nutrition*. 2007 Oct; 86(4):1073–1081.

Cho E, Chen WY, Hunter DJ, Stampfer MJ, Colditz GA, Hankinson SE, Willett WC. "Red meat intake and risk of breast cancer among premenopausal women," *Archives of Internal Medicine*. 2006 Nov 13; 166(20):2253–9.

Cho E, Seddon JM, Rosner B, Willett WC, Hankinson SE. "Prospective study of intake of fruits, vegetables, vitamins, and carotenoids and risk of age-related maculopathy," *Archives of Ophthalmology*. 2004 Jun; 122(6):883–92.

Cordain L, Bryan ED, Melby CL, Smith MJ. "Influence of moderate daily wine consumption on body weight regulation and metabolism in healthy free-living males," *Journal of the American College of Nutrition*. 1997 Apr; 16(2):134–9.

Cordain L, Melby CL, Hamamoto AE, O'Neill DS, Cornier MA, Barakat HA, Israel RG, Hill JO. "Influence of moderate chronic wine consumption on insulin sensitivity and other correlates of syndrome X in moderately obese women," *Metabolism: Clinical and Experimental*. 2000 Nov; 49(11):1473–8.

Djurovic S, Berge KE, Birkenes B, Braaten O, Retterstøl L. "The effect of red wine on plasma leptin levels and vasoactive factors from adipose tissue: A randomized crossover trial," *Alcohol and Alcoholism*. 2007 Nov-Dec; 42(6):525–8. Epub 2007 Aug 1.

Fairfield KM, Hunter DJ, Colditz GA, Fuchs CS, Cramer DW, Speizer FE, Willett WC, Hankinson SE. "A prospective study of dietary lactose and ovarian cancer," *International Journal of Cancer*. 2004 Jun 10; 110(2):271–7.

Flechtner-Mors M, Biesalski HK, Jenkinson CP, Adler G, Ditschuneit HH. "Effects of moderate consumption of white wine on weight loss in overweight and obese subjects," *International Journal of Obesity and Related Metabolic Disorders*. 2004 Nov; 28(11):1420–6.

Gatseva PD, Argirova MD. "Iodine status of children living in areas with high nitrate levels in water," *Archives of Environmental and Occupational Health*. 2005 Nov-Dec; 60(6):317–9.

Ghanta S, Banerjee A, Poddar A, Chattopadhyay S. "Oxidative DNA damage preventive activity and antioxidant potential of *Stevia rebaudiana* (Bertoni) Bertoni, a Natural Sweetener," *Journal of Agricultural and Food Chemistry*. 2007 Dec 26 55(26) 10962–7.

Gregersen S, Jeppesen PB, Holst JJ, Hermansen K. "Antihyperglycemic effects of stevioside in type 2 diabetic subjects," *Metabolism: Clinical and Experimental*. 2004 Jan; 53(1):73–6.

Halkjaer J, Tjønneland A, Thomsen BL, Overvad K, Sørensen TI. "Intake of macronutrients as predictors of 5-y changes in waist circumference," *American Journal of Clinical Nutrition*. 2006 Oct; 84(4):789–97.

Halton TL, Willett WC, Liu S, Manson JE, Albert CM, Rexrode K, Hu FB. "Low-carbohydrate-diet score and the risk of coronary heart disease in women," *New England Journal of Medicine*. 2006 Nov 9; 355(19):1991–2002.

Halton TL, Willett WC, Liu S, Manson JE, Stampfer MJ, Hu FB. "Potato and french fry consumption and risk of type 2 diabetes in women," *American Journal of Clinical Nutrition*. 2006 Feb; 83(2):284–90.

Heymsfield SB, van Mierlo CA, van der Knaap HC, Heo M, Frier HI. "Weight management using a meal replacement strategy: Meta and pooling analysis from six studies," *International Journal of Obesity and Related Metabolic Disorders*. 2003 May; 27(5):537–49.

Humphries P, Pretorius E, Naudé H. "Direct and indirect cellular effects of aspartame on the brain," *European Journal of Clinical Nutrition*. 2008 April 62(4): 451–62.

Hung HC, Joshipura KJ, Jiang R, Hu FB, Hunter D, Smith-Warner SA, Colditz GA, Rosner B, Spiegelman D, Willett WC. "Fruit and vegetable intake and risk of major chronic disease," *Journal of the National Cancer Institute*. 2004 Nov 3; 96(21):1577–84.

Jakszyn P, Gonzalez CA. "Nitrosamine and related food intake and gastric and oesophageal cancer risk: A systematic review of the epidemiological evidence," *World Journal of Gastroenterology*. 2006 Jul 21; 12(27):4296–303.

Kim EH, Willett WC, Colditz GA, Hankinson SE, Stampfer MJ, Hunter DJ, Rosner B, Holmes MD. "Dietary fat and risk of postmenopausal breast cancer in a 20-year follow-up," *American Journal of Epidemiology*. 2006 Nov 15; 164(10):990–7.

Kimura Y, Kono S, Toyomura K, Nagano J, Mizoue T, Moore MA, Mibu R, Tanaka M, Kakeji Y, Maehara Y, Okamura T, Ikejiri K, Futami K, Yasunami Y, Maekawa T, Takenaka K, Ichimiya H, Imaizumi N. "Meat, fish and fat intake in relation to subsite-specific risk of colorectal cancer: The Fukuoka Colorectal Cancer Study," *Cancer Science*. 2007 Apr; 98(4):590–7.

Kuo HW, Wu TN, Yang CY. "Nitrates in drinking water and risk of death from rectal cancer in Taiwan," *Journal of Toxicology and Environmental Health* Part A. 2007 Oct; 70(20):1717–22.

La Rocca C, Mantovani A. "From environment to food: The case of PCB," *Annali dell'Istituto Superiore di Sanità*. 2006; 42(4):410–6.

LeCheminant JD, Jacobsen DJ, Hall MA, Donnelly JE. "A comparison of meal replacements and medication in weight maintenance after weight loss," *Journal of the American College of Nutrition*. 2005 Oct; 24(5):347–53.

Lee JE, Hunter DJ, Spiegelman D, Adami HO, Bernstein L, van den Brandt PA, Buring JE, Cho E, English D, Folsom AR, Freudenheim JL, Gile GG, Giovannucci E, Horn-Ross PL, Leitzmann M, Marshall JR, Männistö S, McCullough ML, Miller AB, Parker AS, Pietinen P, Rodriguez C, Rohan TE, Schatzkin A, Schouten LJ, Willett WC, Wolk A, Zhang SM, Smith-Warner SA. "Intakes of coffee, tea, milk, soda and juice and renal cell cancer in a pooled analysis of 13 prospective studies," *International Journal of Cancer*. 2007 Nov 15; 121(10):2246–53.

Lenoir M, Serre F, Cantin L, Ahmed SH. "Intense sweetness surpasses cocaine reward," *PLoS ONE*. 2007 Aug 1; 2(1):e698.

Lopez-Garcia E, Schulze MB, Manson JE, Meigs JB, Albert CM, Rifai N, Willett WC, Hu FB. "Consumption of (n-3) fatty acids is related to plasma biomarkers of inflammation and endothelial activation in women," *Journal of Nutrition*. 2004 Jul; 134(7):1806–11.

Lopez-Garcia E, Schulze MB, Meigs JB, Manson JE, Rifai N, Stampfer MJ, Willett WC, Hu FB. "Consumption of trans fatty acids is related to plasma biomarkers of inflammation and endothelial dysfunction," *Journal of Nutrition*. 2005 Mar; 135(3):562–6.

Martínez ME, Jacobs ET, Ashbeck EL, Sinha R, Lance P, Alberts DS, Thompson PA. "Meat intake, preparation methods, mutagens and colorectal adenoma recurrence," *Carcinogenesis*. 2007 Sep; 28(9):2019–27. Epub 2007 Aug 8.

Michels KB, Giovannucci E, Chan AT, Singhania R, Fuchs CS, Willett WC. "Fruit and vegetable consumption and colorectal adenomas in the Nurses' Health Study," *Cancer Research*. 2006 Apr 1; 66(7):3942–53.

Mozaffarian D, Pischon T, Hankinson SE, Rifai N, Joshipura K, Willett WC, Rimm EB. "Dietary intake of trans fatty acids and systemic inflammation in women," *American Journal of Clinical Nutrition*. 2004 Apr; 79(4):606–12.

Oh K, Hu FB, Cho E, Rexrode KM, Stampfer MJ, Manson JE, Liu S, Willett WC. "Carbohydrate intake, glycemic index, glycemic load, and dietary fiber in relation to risk of stroke in women," *American Journal of Epidemiology*. 2005 Jan 15; 161(2):161–9.

Oh K, Hu FB, Manson JE, Stampfer MJ, Willett WC. "Dietary fat intake and risk of coronary heart disease in women: 20 years of follow-up of the Nurses' Health Study," *American Journal of Epidemiology*. 2005 Apr 1; 161(7):672–9.

Park Y, Hunter DJ, Spiegelman D, Bergkvist L, Berrino F, van den Brandt PA, Buring JE, Colditz GA, Freudenheim JL, Fuchs CS, Giovannucci E, Goldbohm RA, Graham S, Harnack L, Hartman AM, Jacobs DR Jr, Kato I, Krogh V, Leitzmann MF, McCullough ML, Miller AB, Pietinen P, Rohan TE, Schatzkin A, Willett WC, Wolk A, Zeleniuch-Jacquotte A, Zhang SM, Smith-Warner SA. "Dietary fiber intake and risk of colorectal cancer: a pooled analysis of prospective cohort studies," *Journal of the American Medical Association*. 2005 Dec 14; 294(22):2849–57.

Patel RM, Sarma R, Grimsley E. "Popular sweetner sucralose as a migraine trigger," *Headache*. 2006 Sep; 46(8):1303–4.

Pierce WD, Heth CD, Owczarczyk JC, Russell JC, Proctor SD. "Overeating by young obesity-prone and lean rats caused by tastes associated with low energy foods," *Obesity* (Silver Spring, MD). 2007 Aug; 15(8):1969–79.

Raynor HA, Epstein LH. "Dietary variety, energy regulation, and obesity," *Psychological Bulletin*. 127, (3).

Schulze MB, Manson JE, Willett WC, Hu FB. "Processed meat intake and incidence of type 2 diabetes in younger and middle-aged women," *Diabetologia*. 2003 Nov; 46(11):1465–73. Epub 2003 Oct 24.

Soffritti M, Belpoggi F, Tibaldi E, Esposti DD, Lauriola M. "Life-span exposure to low doses of aspartame beginning during prenatal life increases cancer effects in rats," *Environmental Health Perspectives*. 2007 Sep; 115(9):1293–7.

Tamimi RM, Hankinson SE, Campos H, Spiegelman D, Zhang S, Colditz GA, Willett WC, Hunter DJ. "Plasma carotenoids, retinol, and tocopherols and risk of breast cancer," *American Journal of Epidemiology*. 2005 Jan 15; 161(2):153–60.

Taylor EF, Burley VJ, Greenwood DC, Cade JE. "Meat consumption and risk of breast cancer in the UK Women's Cohort Study," *British Journal of Cancer*. 2007 Apr 10; 96(7):1139–46.

Thomson BM, Nokes CJ, Cressey PJ. "Intake and risk assessment of nitrate and nitrite from New Zealand foods and drinking water," *Food Additives and Contaminants*. 2007 Feb; 24(2):113–21.

Toden S, Bird AR, Topping DL, Conlon MA. "High red meat diets induce greater numbers of colonic DNA double-strand breaks than white meat in rats: Attenuation by high amylose maize starch," *Carcinogenesis*. 2007 Nov; 28(11): 2355–62.

Tsai CJ, Leitzmann MF, Hu FB, Willett WC, Giovannucci EL. "Frequent nut consumption and decreased risk of cholecystectomy in women," *American Journal of Clinical Nutrition*. 2004 Jul; 80(1):76–81.

Tsai CJ, Leitzmann MF, Willett WC, Giovannucci EL. "Fruit and vegetable consumption and risk of cholecystectomy in women," *American Journal of Medicine*. 2006 Sep; 119(9):760–7.

———. "Glycemic load, glycemic index, and carbohydrate intake in relation to risk of cholecystectomy in women," *Gastroenterology*. 2005 Jul; 129(1):105–12.

van Dam RM, Willett WC, Manson JE, Hu FB. "Coffee, caffeine, and risk of type 2 diabetes: A prospective cohort study in younger and middle-aged U.S. women," *Diabetes Care*. 2006 Feb; 29(2):398–403.

Varraso R, Jiang R, Barr RG, Willett WC, Camargo CA Jr. "Prospective study of cured meats consumption and risk of chronic obstructive pulmonary disease in men," *American Journal of Epidemiology*. 2007 Dec; 166(12): 1438–45.

Wadden TA, Butryn ML, Wilson C. "Lifestyle modification for the management of obesity," *Gastroenterology*. 2007 May; 132(6):2226–38.

Wannamethee SG, Shaper AG, Whincup PH. "Alcohol and adiposity: Effects of quantity and type of drink and time relation with meals," *International Journal of Obesity* (London). 2005 Dec; 29(12):1436–44.

Weihrauch MR, Diehl V. "Artificial sweeteners—do they bear a carcinogenic risk?" *Annals of Oncology: Official Journal of the European Society for Medical Oncology/ESMO*. 2004 Oct; 15(10):1460–5.

Westerterp-Plantenga MS, Verwegen CR. "The appetizing effect of an apéritif in overweight and normal-weight humans," *American Journal of Clinical Nutrition*. 1999 Feb; 69(2):205–12.

Willett W. "Lessons from dietary studies in Adventists and questions for the future," *American Journal of Clinical Nutrition*. 2003 Sep; 78(3 Suppl):539S–543S.

Willett WC. "The Mediterranean diet: Science and practice," *Public Health Nutrition*. 2006 Feb; 9(1A):105–10.

Winkelmayer WC, Stampfer MJ, Willett WC, Curhan GC. "Habitual caffeine intake and the risk of hypertension in women," *Journal of the American Medical Association*. 2005 Nov 9; 294(18):2330–5.

Wu K, Giovannucci E, Byrne C, Platz EA, Fuchs C, Willett WC, Sinha R. "Meat mutagens and risk of distal colon adenoma in a cohort of U.S. men," *Cancer Epidemiology, Biomarkers, and Prevention*. A Publication of the American Association for Cancer Research, cosponsored by the American Society of Preventive Oncology. 2006 Jun; 15(6):1120–5.

Zhang SM, Willett WC, Selhub J, Manson JE, Colditz GA, Hankinson SE. "A prospective study of plasma total cysteine and risk of breast cancer," *Cancer Epidemiology, Biomarkers, and Prevention*. 2003 Nov; 12(11 Pt 1):1188–93.

CHAPTER 4

Bell SJ, Goodrick GK. "A functional food product for the management of weight," *Critical Reviews in Food Science and Nutrition*. 2002 Mar; 42(2):163–78.

Birdsall TC. "5-hydroxytryptophan: A clinically-effective serotonin precursor," *Alternative Medicine Reviews*. 1998 Aug; 3(4):271–80.

Bruni O, Ferri R, Miano S, Verrillo E. "L-5-hydroxytryptophan treatment of sleep terrors in children." *European Journal of Pediatrics*. 2004 Jul; 163(7):402–7. Epub 2004 May 14.

Carmichael SL, Shaw GM, Yang W, Abrams B, Lammer EJ. "Maternal stressful life events and risks of birth defects," *Epidemiology*. 2007 May; 18(3):356–61.

Caruso I, Sarzi Puttini P, Cazzola M, Azzolini V. "Double-blind study of 5-hydroxytryptophan versus placebo in the treatment of primary fibromyalgia syndrome," *Journal of International Medical Research*. 1990 May–Jun; 18(3):201–9.

Daily values: http://www.cfsan.fda.gov/~dms/flg-7a.html.

Enstrom JE, Kanim LE, Klein MA. "Vitamin C intake and mortality among a sample of the United States population," *Epidemiology*. 1992 May; 3(3):194–202.

Fairfield KM, Fletcher RH. "Vitamins for chronic disease prevention in adults: Scientific review," *Journal of the American Medical Association*. 2002 Jun 19; 287(23):3116–26.

Fletcher RH, Fairfield KM. "Vitamins for chronic disease prevention in adults: Clinical applications," *Journal of the American Medical Association*. 2002 Jun 19; 287(23): 3127–9.

Goldberg RJ, Katz J. "A meta-analysis of the analgesic effects of omega-3 polyunsaturated fatty acid supplementation for inflammatory joint pain," *Pain*. 2007 May; 129(1–2):210-23. Epub 2007 Mar 1.

Jacobson TA. "Beyond lipids: The role of omega-3 fatty acids from fish oil in the prevention of coronary heart disease," *Current Atherosclerosis Reports*. 2007 Aug; 9(2):145–53.

Kraus VB, Huebner JL, Stabler T, Flahiff CM, Setton LA, Fink C, Vilim V, Clark AG. "Ascorbic acid increases the severity of spontaneous knee osteoarthritis in a guinea pig model," *Arthritis and Rheumatism*. 2004 Jun; 50(6):1822–31.

Lin PY, Su KP. "A meta-analytic review of double-blind, placebo-controlled trials of antidepressant efficacy of omega-3 fatty acids," *Journal of Clinical Psychiatry*. 2007 Jul; 68(7):1056–61.

McAlindon TE. "Nutraceuticals: Do they work and when should we use them?" *Best Practice and Research in Clinical Rheumatology*. 2006 Feb; 20(1):99–115.

McAlindon TE, Biggee BA. "Nutritional factors and osteoarthritis: Recent developments," *Current Opinions in Rheumatology*. 2005 Sep; 17(5):647–52.

Rodríguez-Rodríguez E, Ortega RM, López-Sobaler AM, Aparicio A, Bermejo LM, Marín-Arias LI. "The relationship between antioxidant nutrient intake and cataracts in older people," *International Journal of Vitamin Nutrition Research*. 2006 Nov; 76(6): 359–66.

Sarzi Puttini P, Caruso I. "Primary fibromyalgia syndrome and 5-hydroxy-L-tryptophan: A 90-day open study," *Journal of International Medical Research*. 1992 Apr; 20(2):182–9.

Shirodaria C, Antoniades C, Lee J, Jackson CE, Robson MD, Francis JM, Moat SJ, Ratnatunga C, Pillai R, Refsum H, Neubauer S, Channon KM. "Global improvement of vascular function and redox state with low-dose folic acid: Implications for folate therapy in patients with coronary artery disease," *Circulation*. 2007 May 1; 115(17):2262–70.

Simopoulos AP. "Omega-3 fatty acids and athletics," *Current Sports Medicine Reports*. 2007 Jul; 6(4):230–6.

Wang Y, Hodge AM, Wluka AE, English DR, Giles GG, O'Sullivan R, Forbes A, Cicuttini FM. "Effect of antioxidants on knee cartilage and bone in healthy, middle-aged subjects: A cross-sectional study," *Arthritis Research Therapy*. 2007 Jul 6; 9(4):R66.

Yokoyama T, Date C, Kokubo Y, Yoshiike N, Matsumura Y, Tanaka H. "Serum vitamin C concentration was inversely associated with subsequent 20-year incidence of stroke in a Japanese rural community," *Stroke*. 2000 Oct; 31(10):2287–94. The Shibata study.

Yoshida M, Takashima Y, Inoue M, Iwasaki M, Otani T, Sasaki S, Tsugane S; JPHC Study Group. "Prospective study showing that dietary vitamin C reduced the risk of age-related cataracts in a middle-aged Japanese population," *European Journal of Nutrition*. 2007 Mar; 46(2):118–24.

CHAPTER 5

Arakawa M, Tanaka H, Toguchi H, Shirakawa S, Taira K. "Comparative study on sleep health and lifestyle of the elderly in the urban areas and suburbs of Okinawa," *Psychiatry and Clinical Neurosciences*. 2002 Jun; 56(3):245–6.

Bonnet M, Tancer M, Uhde T, Yeragani VK. "Effects of caffeine on heart rate and QT variability during sleep," *Depression and Anxiety*. 2005; 22(3):150–5.

Chilcott LA, Shapiro CM. "The socioeconomic impact of insomnia. An overview," *Pharmacoeconomics*. 1996; 10 (Suppl) 1:1–14.

Drake CL, Jefferson C, Roehrs T, Roth T. "Stress-related sleep disturbance and polysomnographic response to caffeine," *Sleep Medicine*. 2006 Oct; 7(7):567–72. Epub 2006 Sep 22.

Eichling PS, Sahni J. "Menopause related sleep disorders," *Journal of Clinical Sleep Medicine*. 2005 Jul 15; 1(3):291–300.

Gögenur I, Middleton B, Kristiansen VB, Skene DJ, Rosenberg J. "Disturbances in melatonin and core body temperature circadian rhythms after minimal invasive surgery," *Acta Anaesthesiologica Scandinavica*. 2007 Sep; 51(8):1099–106.

Goto A, Yasumura S, Nishise Y, Sakihara S. "Association of health behavior and social role with total mortality among Japanese elders in Okinawa, Japan," *Aging Clinical and Experimental Research*. 2003 Dec; 15(6):443–50.

Haimov I, Hadad BS, Shurkin D. "Visual cognitive function: Changes associated with chronic insomnia in older adults," *Journal of Gerontology in Nursing*. 2007 Oct; 33(10): 32–41.

Harvey AG, Sharpley AL, Ree MJ, Stinson K, Clark DM. "An open trial of cognitive therapy for chronic insomnia," *Behavioral Research Therapy*. 2007 Oct; 45(10):2491–501. Epub 2007 Apr 22.

Humphries P, Pretorius E, Naudé H. "Direct and indirect cellular effects of aspartame on the brain," *European Journal of Clinical Nutrition*. 2008 Apr; (214): 451–62.

Kadono M, Hasegawa G, Shigeta M, Nakazawa A, Ueda M, Fukui M, Yoshikawa T, Nakamura N. "Joint effect of alcohol and usual sleep duration on the risk of dysglycemia," *Sleep*. 2007 Oct 1; 30(10):1341–7.

Karasek M. "Melatonin, human aging, and age-related diseases," *Experimental Gerontology.* 2004 Nov–Dec; 39(11–12):1723–9.

Killgore WD, Kahn-Greene ET, Lipizzi EL, Newman RA, Kamimori GH, Balkin TJ. "Sleep deprivation reduces perceived emotional intelligence and constructive thinking skills," *Sleep Medicine.* 2007 Aug. Epub ahead of print.

Kimata H. "Laughter elevates the levels of breast-milk melatonin," *Journal of Psychosomatic Research.* 2007 Jun; 62(6):699–702.

———. "Viewing humorous film improves nighttime wakening in children with atopic dermatitis," *Indian Pediatrics.* 2007 Apr; 44(4):281–5.

Knutson KL, Spiegel K, Penev P, Van Cauter E. "The metabolic consequences of sleep deprivation," *Sleep Medicine Reviews.* 2007 Jun; 11(3):163–78. Epub 2007 Apr 17.

Kondo M, Tokura H, Wakamura T, Hyun KJ, Tamotsu S, Morita T, Oishi T. "Physiological significance of cyclic changes in room temperature around dusk and dawn for circadian rhythms of core and skin temperature, urinary 6-hydroxymelatonin sulfate, and waking sensation just after rising." *Journal of Physiological Anthropology.* 2007 Jun; 26(4):429-36.

Laposky AD, Bass J, Kohsaka A, Turek FW. "Sleep and circadian rhythms: Key components in the regulation of energy metabolism," *FEBS Letters.* 2007 Aug 14; 582(1):142–151.

Luciano M, Zhu G, Kirk KM, Gordon SD, Heath AC, Montgomery GW, Martin NG. " 'No thanks, it keeps me awake' ": the genetics of coffee-attributed sleep disturbance," *Sleep.* 2007 Oct 1; 30(10):1378–86.

Palma BD, Gabriel A Jr, Colugnati FA, Tufik S. "Effects of sleep deprivation on the development of autoimmune disease in an experimental model of systemic lupus erythematosus," *American Journal of Physiology: Regularity, Integrative and Comparative Physiology.* 2006 Nov; 291(5):R1527–32.

Paterson LM, Wilson SJ, Nutt DJ, Hutson PH, Ivarsson M. "A translational, caffeine-induced model of onset insomnia in rats and healthy volunteers," *Psychopharmacology* (Berlin). 2007 May; 191(4):943–50. Epub 2007 Jan 16.

Penev PD. "Sleep deprivation and energy metabolism: To sleep, perchance to eat?" *Current Opinion in Endocrinology, Diabetes, and Obesity.* 2007 Oct; 14(5):374–81.

Rupp TL, Acebo C, Carskadon MA. "Evening alcohol suppresses salivary melatonin in young adults," *Chronobiology International*. 2007; 24(3):463–70.

Rupp TL, Acebo C, Van Reen E, Carskadon MA. "Effects of a moderate evening alcohol dose. I: sleepiness," *Alcoholism Clinical and Experimental Research*. 2007 Aug; 31(8):1358–64. Epub 2007 Jun 5.

Uezu E, Taira K, Tanaka H, Arakawa M, Urasakii C, Toguchi H, Yamamoto Y, Hamakawa E, Shirakawa S. "Survey of sleep-health and lifestyle of the elderly in Okinawa," *Psychiatry and Clinical Neurosciences*. 2000 Jun; 54(3):311–3.